"Over years of practice I have observed the pain and suffering of my colitis patients who are on conventional medical therapy. High dosages of immuno-suppressants, such as prednisone and like products, are commonly given, resulting in effects ranging from serious to life-threatening. This only suppresses the symptoms temporarily. Disease typically later manifests again, with even more severe and bothersome symptoms.

"I was very impressed with David's Natural Hygiene approach to healing ulcerative colitis and Crohn's disease, outlined in his book *Self Healing Colitis & Crohn's*. Healthy since 1984 after a severe 8-year bout with ulcerative colitis, he himself is living proof that his program works. I support his approach one hundred percent and believe it is the only way of healing colitis and almost all other health problems, and, therefore, I recommend it to every one of my clients. The results are always good because the diet is our natural biological diet, is nontoxic, nutritionally superior, satisfying, and since only the body's own wisdom can heal itself, the Natural Hygiene approach makes perfect sense."

Zarin Azar, M.D., Gastroenterologist
Los Angeles, California <drzarinazar@yahoo.com>

≈

"David has exhibited uncommon dedication to helping people become well over the twelve years I have known him. Like David, in my practice I see long-lasting results when a patient embraces a detoxification program and adopts a healthful lifestyle with a vegan diet. David's recovery from severe ulcerative colitis, his studies in nutrition and physiology, and his consistent results have given him unique expertise in self-healing. In *Self Healing Colitis & Crohn's* we have the blueprint for overcoming IBD."

Terri Su, M.D.
Santa Rosa, California

≈

"I know of no physician who is not reluctant to prescribe corticosteroids or advise surgery for the treatment of inflammatory bowel disease, and yet they are the mainstays of traditional therapy. In *Self Healing Colitis & Crohn's* is a clear and detailed healing plan that eschews both and offers a program based on the author's personal experience and extensive research. It deserves our grateful attention."

Robert F. Lally Jr., M.D.
Friday Harbor, Washington

"Ulcerative colitis is a debilitating disease that has long been regarded as untreatable. For many patients, the illness has therefore meant considerable suffering and the end of a normally functioning life. Thanks to David Klein, this need no longer be true. *Self Healing Colitis & Crohn's* is an insightful and compassionate book by a leading nutritionist who suffered from this crippling disease, cured himself and has since gone on to become a pioneer in effective nutritional counseling. It is a must read for anyone who wants an active role in restoring himself or herself to health."

A. William Menzin, M.D., M.Sc., M.P.H.
Department of Psychiatry, Harvard Medical School (retired)
Former Consultant to the World Health Organization (WHO)
Princeton, New Jersey

❧

"Dr. David Klein's *Self Healing Colitis & Crohn's* demystifies the secrets of the innate natural health processes, by which the body possesses the power to heal itself. A Hygienic Doctor and former victim of ulcerative colitis, Dr. Klein is the leading modern-day pioneer and authority on the self-healing principles of colitis and Crohn's disease. He is living proof that the body can cure itself and maintain its natural, pristine health when the causes of disease are removed and it is allowed to perform its magical healing-dance of life."

Paul Fanny, Ph.D., H.D.
President of the University of Natural Health
Hookset, New Hampshire

❧

"When it comes to self-healing, my dear friend Dave Klein has been there and done that, like very few have ever done. His depth of understanding of the issues involved in the causes and healing of bowel disease is only matched by his compassion for current sufferers. There is no reason for anyone else to write on this topic because Dave has already perfected the healing process. Like the law of gravity, his program works first time, every time. Put it to work for you and suffer no more."

Douglas N. Graham, D.C.
Author of *The 80/10/10 Diet*
Key Largo, Florida

Self Healing Colitis & Crohn's

3rd Edition

by David Klein, Ph.D.

Hygienic Doctor

Director, Colitis & Crohn's Health Recovery Center

Self Healing Colitis & Crohn's
by David Klein, Ph.D.
© 1993, 2005, 2006, 2008, 2009 David Klein, Ph.D.
Third Edition, June, 2009

Colitis & Crohn's Health Recovery Center
Post Box 256
Sebastopol, CA 95473 USA

www.colitis-crohns.com
www.colitiscurebook.com
dave@colitis-crohns.com
(877) 740-6082; (707) 829-0462

Cover photo by David Klein

Book design by Robert Marcus Graphics, Sebastopol, California

$23.95
ISBN 978-0-9717526-4-1

Printed in Canada

Self Healing
Colitis & Crohn's

3rd Edition

TABLE OF CONTENTS

SECTION 5 – YOUR NEW HEALTHFUL LIFESTYLE

SECTION 6 – INSPIRATION

SECTION 7 – APPENDICES

FIGURES

ACKNOWLEDGEMENTS

Special thanks go to Dr. Edward Bauman and Dr. Griselda Blazey for helping me to craft my original report on this theme; to my dear mother Doris and friends Jenifer Ransom and Johanna Zee for their careful copy editing; and to Robert Marcus for his enlivening publishing design work.

DEDICATIONS

To Charlie Abel, Dr. Iraj Afshar, Dr. Zarin Azar, Don Bennett, Dr. Alec Burton, Dr. T. Colin Campbell, Donna Dixon-Mannios, Dr. Lyudmila Emilova, Dr. Paul Fanny, Dr. T. C. Fry, Dr. Laurence Galant, Dr. Roe Gallo, Dr. Alan Goldhamer, Dr. Douglas Graham, Professor Rozalind Graham, Sylvester Graham, Roger Haeske, John Henao, Frieda Ireland, Dr. Susan Smith Jones, John Kohler, Morris Krok, Dr. Robert F. Lally Jr., Nick Ledger, Shannon Leone, Dr. Mamiko Matsuda, Dr. A. William Menzin, Dr. Samuel Mielcarski, Dennis Nelson, Florence Nightingale, Karen Ranzi, Dr. Frank Sabatino, Bradley Saul, Dr. Gina Shaw, Dr. Herbert M. Shelton, Dr. Robert Sniadach, Dr. Terri Su, Grace Swanson, Dr. John Tilden, Dr. Timothy Trader, Sydney Vallentyne, Dr. Vivian V. Vetrano, Don Weaver and Johanna Zee, Ph.D. for holding up the light and showing the way.

To my parents, Doris and Edward, for their loving support.

To my greatest instinctual teachers: Whisky, Greystoke, Simba and Carmella.

To the magnificent self-healing power within us all.

FOREWORD

Colitis and Crohn's disease (C&C) are inflammatory bowel illnesses characterized by distressful bowel function. "Itis" means inflammation. The body's intelligence system creates inflammation just as it creates fevers. Inflammation is an escalated healing action in which harmful toxic matter is being broken down and neutralized for elimination at a "feverish pace." Toxins in the body cause the body to enact inflammation for purification.

The body enacts disease processes, such as C&C, in response to systemic toxicosis, i.e., when the body is overloaded with toxins. A bowel with C&C is overloaded with toxic fecal matter which saturates the tissues and typically impairs elimination. C&C symptoms are "housecleaning" processes. The more acutely toxic the body and the more vital the body's nerve energy, the more intense the self-cleansing/healing process. C&C symptoms will diminish as the body detoxifies, which requires that the ingestion of toxic, indigestible foodstuffs be discontinued and a health-promoting diet and lifestyle be adopted.

Medical researchers, doctors and nurses mistakenly believe that the body's inflammation response is an "autoimmune" phenomenon. That is incorrect and illogical. The body only works to heal itself and never creates any physiological process that would harm itself. When the body is inflamed, the body is acting to break down, neutralize and eliminate toxins, not healthy tissue. And some researchers believe that bacteria cause ulcers. This is also incorrect. Bacteria consume wastes and assist in elimination. They are not capable of causing bodily actions. Ulcers are an open outlet for the elimination of toxins from the bloodstream. The body intelligently resorts to creating ulcers when the load of toxins in the bloodstream is too great for the body to neutralize and eliminate, via the immune system and inflammation alone. Both inflammation and ulceration are manifestations of detoxification and healing. They are the body's way of "curing" itself; inflammation and ulceration are self-healing processes in action. In order to self-heal, one must understand and trust all self-healing processes.

The symptoms of C&C may be considered as a warning that the results of inappropriate lifestyle and dietary habits have reached a stage requiring that immediate changes be made. C&C are most common in societies, such as the West, where meat is a major part of the diet and stress from fast-paced modern lifestyles is prevalent.

The Crohn's and Colitis Foundation (CCFA) estimates there are 1.5 million IBD sufferers in the United States. The Crohn's and Colitis Foundation of Canada's estimate for Canada is 170,000. The European Federation of Crohn's and Ulcerative Colitis Association's estimate for Europe is 1.2 million. The Australian

Crohn's and Colitis Foundation's estimate for Australia is 61,000. CCFA reports a 10-fold increase in IBD in the United States, Europe and Japan since World War II.

Medical authorities state that prolonged suffering with C&C can result in cancer. Colorectal cancer ranks number three in cancer-related mortalities in the United States (behind lung and prostate cancers). There are two basic forms of inflammatory bowel diseases:

1. Colitis is an inflammation of the colon. Local symptoms may include diarrhea, mucous formation, bleeding, constipation, abdominal cramps, spasms, colon disfigurement, flatulence, abdominal and rectal pain, fevers and stomach distress. Related non-local symptoms can be many, including weight loss, emotional distress, headaches, sleeping difficulties, general weakness and rapid aging. The use of anti-inflammatory, antibiotic and immunosuppressant medications, while sometimes temporarily suppressing symptoms, always have effects which contribute further to the devitalization of the person's health. Drugs are toxic and enervating; the body expends precious energy as it works to get rid of them.

Colitis may advance into ulcerative colitis which is characterized by inflammation and ulceration(s) of the colon. Symptoms can include all of those listed above plus painful ulcerations in the colon wall which can both perforate the colon and/or become cancerous.

2. Crohn's disease, or regional enteritis, is an inflammation of any portion of the alimentary canal. It usually affects the lower section of the small intestine—the ileum—giving rise to the name "ileitis." Symptoms are typically similar to those for colitis.

C&C, if not treated wholistically, typically has a life-ruining effect. Surgical removal of the colon is often considered by the medical establishment to be a standard treatment for chronic cases of colitis and ulcerative colitis. In the past decade, some (but too few) medical doctors have begun to recognize that specific dietary changes can lead to an improvement in C&C. It is prudent for persons with C&C, even in advanced cases, to get opinions from wholistically-trained and experienced health practitioners before submitting to drug therapy and surgery. Most, if not all, colon surgeries are unnecessary.

The way to overcome C&C is to: 1. stop poisoning and enervating the body with drugs, harmful foods and lifestyle stressors, 2. adopt a restful healing program fulfilling our basic health needs, including eating our natural biological diet while allowing the organism to complete the healing process. The body cannot simultaneously accomplish healing while poisons are ingested. Harmful foods include: meat and dairy from any animal source, processed grain products, heated fatty foods including oils, irritants such as spices, salt and onions and all processed "junk foods" and beverages, including coffee.

The Natural Hygiene self-healing plan with the Vegan Healing diet taught in this book work because they are based on the immutable laws governing human biology and physiology. When we discontinue unhealthful practices and provide the requisites of health, eating our natural biological diet, the body will only improve itself, reversing disease, completely healing and creating new health. As long as the dietary and lifestyle factors which cause enervation and toxemia are avoided, wellness will last and C&C will not return.

The body is designed or "programmed" for perfect self-healing. It will regenerate every cell in the organism, break down strictures and scar tissue in the bowel, autolyze polyps and, in most cases, even tumors, and restore health when given the proper care and lifestyle program, as taught herein.

The author recommends and the body demands that people with C&C take a restful sabbatical of three months or more in order to give the body and mind the rest needed for effective self-healing. If you are unable to do this, do the best you can and take as much rest and extra sleep as is possible.

NOTES TO READER

1. Throughout this book "C&C" is used to refer to colitis and Crohn's disease.

2. Some duly noted sections of this manuscript were taken from various magazine articles and booklets authored and published by the late great Hygienic educators, Dr. T. C. Fry and Dr. Herbert M. Shelton. Their works were uncopyrighted offerings intended for the benefit of humanity; as their work saved my life and many others' lives and their families have permitted me their use, it is my great privilege and duty to pass them on. Some other sections were reprinted with the permission of living authors who are my colleagues. The sections written by authors other than, or with, myself are presented in italics. The sections where the author is not named were written by myself.

3. Many will question and prematurely discount this healing plan as being "unscientific," i.e., not medically validated. That line of thinking is illogical. The modern medical establishment is not the authority on what is scientific and healthful. Modern medical men and women typically either ignore or "shoot down" natural healing approaches. For the most part, modern medicine is interested in medicating and surgically altering patients. Therefore, this information has not interested medical people. Factual truth stands on its own. This program is entirely scientific. That which is scientific yields consistently positive results and is authentically good. My 1,000-plus clients who have healed are not aberrations or anomalies—they are real evidence that this approach works, as is my recovery and 25 years of superb health. I have seen this approach work in over 99% of the clients who have properly implemented the plan. I am trained as a scientist and educator. I hold a Bachelor of Science degree in engineering and have 10 years of experience in engineering. I also have 25 years of experience in health science and hold a Ph.D. in Natural Health and Healing. I have lived over 25 years in disease-free health, beyond what one gastroenterologist forecasted was possible. Scientifically speaking, the results speak for themselves and are conclusively positive. The body is obviously able to consistently and naturally self-heal C&C under the proper conditions. Skepticism is understandable. I was was once there! Skeptics are welcome to contact me to discuss the healing and lifestyle approach presented herein.

4. Many will reject the natural vegan dietary approach espoused herein without studying the facts and contacting me, presuming that:
   A. It is nutritionally insufficient, especially in protein, calcium and calories.
   B. Animal meat is essential to health.
   C. Their blood type or genetics dispose them to require meat.
   D. They crave protein and there isn't enough in vegan foods.

E. They cannot tolerate fruit.

F. The diet is too restrictive.

G. Extreme, permanent weight loss and physical weakness will result.

H. They won't feel satisfied and will miss meat and other favorite foods.

I. Others are able to "get away" with eating omnivorous diets with meat, so they should, too.

J. They won't be able to cope socially.

K. They do not believe they can change their habits.

All of those claims are based on misinformation, unfounded assumptions or pessimistic, self-limiting projections. Solid empirical science conclusively demonstrates that there is no lack of any one nutrient in the fruit-based vegan diet espoused herein which is essential to health, while it is animal foods, especially meat, which cause inflammatory bowel disease. Also, the Vegan Diet recommended herein supplies superior nutrition, as consistently confirmed by full-panel blood tests. Furthermore, foods outside of its realm are unnecessary; they cause myriad problems and most lead to C&C; this diet eliminates all of the dietary factors which cause C&C and includes the most healthful diet program for humans.

Fruit is our most naturally healthful food and, when eaten in accordance with the specific guidelines presented herein, is the primary essential food for healing C&C and maintaining good health. When humans correctly eat the original diet for which they were designed, the inevitable result is healing and optimal health. As evidenced by hundreds of thousands people who have actualized superb health on vegan diets similar or identical to the one advised herein, this approach is conclusively valid. We do not experience deprivation or dissatisfaction on this diet because we are eating the foods which we were designed to eat and thrive on, and from which we were naturally designed to derive true pleasure. The result of following this plan is a surprising sense of satisfaction and wellness as we are more thoroughly nourished than ever before, eating a diet of only nutritious foods.

Before dismissing this approach, it is my wish that people try it for three or more months and obtain appropriate counseling in order to make judgments based on personal experience, not on preconceived, self-limiting beliefs which are unfounded. An inquisitive mind and willingness to question one's beliefs and try an approach which is unconventional are traits which will serve everyone well when the conventional ways of approaching diseases do not work. Those who are able to think "outside the box" and imagine their optimal state of health in relation to the natural order of life are the ones who succeed in overcoming C&C. Solving the C&C problem is a matter of thinking for oneself and aligning with our natural instincts—not technology, medical science, modern conventional dietetics or any healing arts involving remedies. The diet and lifestyle plan presented herein has proven to be the only approach that works because it is based on an accurate understanding of anatomy and the laws of physiology and biology, as borne out by countless successful results. Personal experience is the only way to prove all this true. With appropriate application, the happy truth will be revealed.

5. If you began this program while you are pregnant, continue it and get as much extra rest as possible—this healthful living program is the best thing for mother and child and the quickest route to health.

6. If you are concerned about beginning this program while you are on medications, it is prudent to proceed with the program while following your physician's recommendations regarding medication dosage. The Vegan Healing Diet will only promote health; there is no reason to postpone its implementation.

7. If you are concerned about the suitability of this diet program for children, it is certainly appropriate and offers complete and superior nutrition. Starches, meat and dairy foods including cow's milk should not be fed to infants and children with C&C. For infants or children under age four, human breast milk is recommended in conjunction with the Vegan Healing Diet.

8. To successfully apply the teachings herein, it is necessary to fully understand the subject matter. It is therefore recommended that this book be read several if not numerous times and professional guidance be obtained.

1
INTRODUCTION

1.1

WE POSSESS SELF-HEALING BODIES AND WERE NOT MEANT TO SUFFER!

We were not designed or born into this world to be sick with inflamed bowels. Our genes do not cause us to become sick with inflammatory bowel disease, but, rather, our diets, lifestyles and thoughts are the causes—and they can all be corrected and we can and will heal if we implement the right healing plan.

The body is a perfectly designed self-healing organism. Bowel inflammation is not a runaway problem but a sign that the body has been harmed and is vigorously attempting to heal itself, and it will gratefully do so if the causes of disease are discontinued and the biological requisites of health are provided. The solution to bowel disease is to identify the harmful factors, discontinue them and implement a new healthful lifestyle with health-promoting practices. A few million people have done this, overcoming all kinds of debilitating disease conditions, including inflammatory and irritable bowel diseases—and so can you!

Contrary to conventional belief, there is no mystery behind why we become sick and there is no lack of understanding of how to overcome disease, heal and rejuvenate. Those who have applied the Natural Hygiene system of self-healthcare have overcome diseases which include colitis, ulcerative colitis, Crohn's disease, ileitis, irritable bowel syndrome and every other gastrointestinal malady humanity has ever experienced, including some cases of cancer.

Herein is a specialized Hygienic healing plan for those who wish to overcome bowel disease and create disease-free vigorous health. All of this information is not based upon theories or anything that the author invented. Hygienic healing, i.e., cooperating with nature, removing the causes of disease and fulfilling our biological requisites for health, is the way that all creatures have always healed and recovered their health. By deeply delving into these new teachings, letting go of erroneous beliefs, and embracing a new naturally healthful course of action, anyone can dramatically improve his or her condition, and most can go on to master their health and avoid inflammatory bowel problems for the rest of their lives. With proper understanding, help and passionate intention, the goal of disease-free health can be achieved. It takes dedication, work and patience, but it only gets better and better when one immerses oneself in it mind, body and soul. I know—I did it!

In 1984 I began a recovery from the devastating effects of almost nine previous years of ulcerative colitis, which began when I was 17 years old. During my illness, I ate my usual meat and bread-based diet (the "Standard American Diet," or "SAD"), and was under only medical guidance which consisted of examinations by gastroenterologists, hospitalizations and drug treatment. All of the seven gastroenterologists I saw told me that diet was not a factor in my illness, that there was no known cause of ulcerative colitis, and the only available treatments were drugs, and if they didn't work, then surgical removal of my colon was the best alternative.

In the last year of my illness, my colon was ravaged with ulcerations, my health was in ruins, and surgical removal of my colon was recommended. At that time, I was consulting a nutrition guidance counselor who had a doctorate in Natural Hygiene. He recommended that I follow a natural diet essentially of only fruits and vegetables (a Natural Hygiene program, which has since been popularized by the best-selling book *Fit For Life,* written by Harvey and Marilyn Diamond). At first I rejected this advice; however, I slowly began to "clean up" my diet. Still, my colon was inflamed and ulcerated. In October of 1984, just after a gastroenterologist recommended a colostomy (surgical removal of my colon), my fortune changed as one night my studies led to a profound understanding of how dietary change could help transform my health. I saw the value of eating the diet which early man originally ate, and which our digestive physiology was designed for: mostly fruits, with some vegetables, seeds and nuts, and no animal products. The next day I changed from the SAD to a natural diet of mostly uncooked fruits and vegetables. I also ceased using medicines for good (I had been on low dosages at the time). The result was astonishing, but typical: my colon immediately and rapidly began healing up, and totally and permanently healed up within four weeks.

From there I went on to rejuvenate my severely depleted body. Since the day I changed my diet, I have immersed myself in the study of natural healing and worked on completely rebuilding my health without the use of any medications or other unnatural intervention.

Today I am in excellent health and fitness at age 51, and feel like a teenager. I am very passionate about teaching others with C&C how to regain their health by making sensible dietary and lifestyle changes because I believe that all C&C suffers deserve the same chance to learn about the body's innate ability to heal itself naturally. If you need inspiration to get going and guidance to heal and become well, it is my pleasure to help.

Yours in health,

David Klein, Ph.D.
Sebastopol, California

1.2
SUMMARY

Colitis and Crohn's diseases (C&C) are primarily caused by dietary and other lifestyle stressors. C&C are endemic to cultures where muscle meats and refined foods are eaten as a major portion of the diet and lifestyles have significant stress levels. Animal meats, as well as cooked oils and refined wheat products, are largely indigestible; they poison the bowel as they decompose, acidifying the entire organism and overwhelming the immune and elimination systems, leading to inflammation and distress. Colon and intestinal inflammation are an indication that the body is attempting to purify itself of accumulated toxic matter and heal itself. Inflammation is always the body's intelligent action/response to purify itself of harmful, toxic, irritating poisons and wastes. The healing action is impeded and diseased condition is perpetuated or exacerbated if one continues an improper diet and harmful drug therapy. In view of the evidence showing how countless people have resolved their C&C by changing to a whole foods, vegan diet, and by incorporating stress management techniques, it is best to approach C&C in a wholistic context through dietary and lifestyle changes. A wholistic approach to overcoming C&C should include health education and the implementation of a health-promoting program which includes: 1. a whole foods vegan (no animal-derived foods) diet and juicing; 2. extra sleep and complete rest (a sabbatical from work or school); 3. proper exercise; 4. health counseling; 5. peer support; and 6. medical cooperation. The body is a self-healing organism which will heal when harmful practices are discontinued and healthful practices are implemented. This book details the basic physiological and lifestyle principles which are proven to result not in remission of symptoms but in lasting health. When the causes of disease are removed, health will ensue under the proper care. This is fact, not theory. This book presents no theories and only the happy truth about the magnificent restorative power of the body when it is cared for in a manner which is consonant with our natural biological mandates. By cooperating with nature and changing our injurious lifestyle habits, we'll enjoy a blossoming of health and spirit. This program takes work and discipline, but the better we feel the easier it becomes, on our way to a wonderful life free of suffering and full of happiness and wellness.

1.3
ADVISORY

I, David Klein, am not a medical doctor. I do not diagnose, treat or advise in medical areas. I am an Hygienic Doctor with a Ph.D. in Natural Health and Healing from the University of Natural Health. I am also a state-certified Nutrition Educator, educated, trained and legally certified in counseling people in matters of nutrition, health and healing by the state licensed Bauman College in Penngrove, California. It is my goal to help people safely and permanently heal and become healthy and happy. I can work in concert with medical doctors.

This book is strictly for educational purposes. This book is not a treatment plan nor a personalized healing plan; healing plans must be personalized via individual consultation because each individual has specific needs. The reader is advised to thoroughly study this book and obtain proper professional nutritional and health counseling before making any changes in his or her diet and/or approach to caring for oneself or others. In order to safely and effectively self-heal inflammatory bowel illness, I suggest proper nutritional and health counseling and guidance plus complete rest in all cases.

Any actions taken by the reader, caretaker of persons with inflammatory bowel illness, and/or recipient, and any consequential results from such actions are the sole responsibility of the reader, caretaker and/or recipient. The author is in no way responsible for the recipient's or his/her caretaker's actions and results. Self-healing is safe and effective when one is correctly educated and when correct actions are properly implemented. I recommend gradual health-supportive changes in one's regime. I wish you and yours good health.

2
SELF-HEALING

2.1

Understanding Your Self-Healing Powers

by Dr. T. C. Fry

The Immense Wisdom and Providence of the Body

The human body is possessed of intelligence and powers of an order that is incomprehensible to our intellects. While many humans are vain and will not admit to an inability to know and understand, let's face it: we are all finite in our capacities. We cannot comprehend the concept of infinity, and we are mystified by many simple realities of existence.

From miseducation, ignorance, vanity, authoritarianism, and sheer arrogance amongst our professionals flow incorrect and disastrous actions that brutalize those whom they profess to serve. From intellectual wisdom and understanding flow humility, kindness and other humane virtues. Wisdom recognizes our finite nature and admits to ignorance, an act of humility. Humility does not stifle the innate drive to seek knowledge. Rather, humility is born of a realization that spurs the quest for greater wisdom. True wisdom motivates us to continual exploration and improvement.

This treatise treats an area largely unexplored and uncharted. When we view the vastness of the incredible multitude of faculties possessed by the human body, we must stand in awe of the enormous intelligence displayed in each of the quintillions of processes conducted within the body daily. We must stand in wonderment and awe at the precision we observe. We cannot help but conclude that the body operates on principles that manifest the reign of law and order within the organic realm. We must observe that we are constituted of such an order as to comply in every act with the universal laws of existence.

We want to charge you with an overwhelming realization of the enormity of innate intelligence—of inherent body wisdom that exceeds by thousands of times the intellectual powers of which we arrogantly boast. So vast is this innate intelligence that it is positively staggering. The immensity of inborn intelligence is not an easy subject to present. Very few studies touch upon this subject. However, we can delineate and point out some of the many manifestations of inherent body wisdom.

In this treatise you will become aware of an internal providence that should be respected. So great are our body endowments that you should adopt this attitude:

never interfere with the vital domain. You cannot possibly help it—you can only harm it. All the knowledge and wisdom of civilization to date do not equal the intelligence exhibited by the operations of a single cell within the body! The best you can do is to order the external environment to make it more favorable for the organism. The only thing you can do for the body is to leave it intelligently alone! It knows what it is doing and how! You don't!

Providence is the ability to anticipate needs and provide for them. This providence may be instinctual, as in the case of the bear that stores tremendous amounts of fat in preparation for hibernation, or of the squirrel that stashes nuts, acorns and seeds, or it may be due to acquired wisdom, as in the case of humans who store foods during plenitude in preparation for the season of scarcity.

The body is always provident. All providence exhibits wisdom. The immensity of the wisdom exhibited in all things so overwhelms the human intellect that many often retreat into the comfort of some all-encompassing outlook that tranquilizes them so that they see no mandate to inquire, assess and understand how their actions undermine their well-being.

In studying this program, you are undertaking to delve into life's provisions sufficiently to ascertain a valid course for uplifting yourself and fellow-beings to the utmost possibilities. Wisdom is really a difficult word to assess and define. It can be said to be all-knowing and all-understanding within a given sphere. Wisdom is at once the comprehension of a matter in both depth and breadth. It is an expertise or mastery that enables the possessor to pursue a correct course of action.

In pursuing this study, we must not confuse inherent wisdom or intelligence with intellect and acquired wisdom. The ability to cogitate and think is a property of the conscious intellect. It involves wisdom and intelligence of a different order than the wisdom of the body. For example, if you bite into a luscious apple, the whole system is coursed with delight. If you bite into an apple that has been injected with a solution of caustic soda, you'll immediately recognize the danger, begin spitting and sputtering and run for water to dilute and remove the deadly poison that contacted your mouth tissues. Rejection of toxic matters is just as natural as delighting in beneficent materials and influences.

The Body is Self-Healing

This is self-evident. We observe it in many ways. We see a broken bone knit itself. We see cuts and abrasions heal. We see bruises heal. But most of us, willing to accept that which we readily see, do not believe that the body has sufficient power within to overcome ailments not involving injury. The vital innate healing force is operative at all times. It heals all reparable body injuries and maladies. If the body cannot repair itself, it is irreparable. A tremendous amount of abuse must be heaped upon the body to reach such a low state that it cannot heal itself. At this low state, death is inevitable.

The body works at all times to keep itself in a high-functioning state. It continually works to keep itself pure and as free as possible of toxic wastes. It is endowed with equipment for ejecting foreign material from the vital domain. A body fettered by retained toxic matters and polluted with unwelcome substances from without cannot function at a high level. If the body becomes overburdened, it disables itself through what are called "acute diseases" to hasten the processes of purification and repair. Under the disabled condition, the body marshals its resources to concentrate on internal cleansing and repair of damaged tissue.

All this takes place of the body's own volition, and the best we can do is cooperate. We should take a complete rest so that the body may not be hampered in its endeavors. We should cease all activity, even that of eating. Bed rest in a sunny and airy room with only pure water will greatly facilitate the body's work—you cease to expend energies so that your body may have more.

Nothing inside or outside of nature can substitute for body wisdom. Nothing inside or outside of nature can assume or substitute for body functions. While an ailing body bespeaks a grossly abused body, it will, nevertheless, restore itself to health if the causes of its illness are removed and conditions instituted that permit body restorative activities. If you can see the obvious; that is, that the body is in all cases self-healing, you will: 1. never abuse the temple of your being; and 2. if you suffer from past abuses, not in any way interfere with the body but, under a condition of complete rest, give it command of your energies and resources so that it can more efficiently and quickly repair itself.

Common colds, skin rashes, acne, vomiting, headaches, sinusitis, inflammations and fevers, so-called influenza and a long list of other disabling and frustrating affections are self-healing processes. It is a mistake to try to "cure" them, for they are themselves just that, "curing" processes. But if we do violate the laws of our being, then we must restore health by giving inner body intelligence and powers the opportunity to do so. To try to "cure" a "curing process" is wrong and can cause untold miseries. It adds injury to injury. If a man is repairing a fence and you bludgeon him, he must not only stop fence-mending but contend with a new and more life-threatening enemy.

If your body is repairing itself and you resort to drugs (so-called medicines) that poison the body and so lower its vital powers that it can no longer conduct the reparative process, then your body will remain filled with the offending internal filth, and function will be that much more impaired. When your body is poisoned, the reduction of its vital activities will become readily evident because the symptoms of the reparative process often disappear—the fence-mending has ceased. For instance, a heroin addict's body will start trying to repair itself after being reasonably freed of the heroin. The reparative process is debilitating and pain-wracking. The heroin addict chooses to renarcotize his body with more heroin poison rather than suffer the reparative process. Thus, so-called "withdrawal symptoms," which are really reparative measures, disappear after renewed poisoning. The same process occurs with addicts to the narcotic habits of tobacco and alcohol. Headaches, pains, swellings, etc. are evidences or symptoms of healing processes being conducted by the body. Take a poison (such as aspirin) and you devitalize the body so that it stops the body's mending process, and the symptoms disappear.

If you become ill, do not fight the illness by trying to "remedy" or "cure" it. All such efforts are the same as assaulting the fence repairman. Instead, go to bed in a warm, sunlit room with fresh flowing air. Drink only pure water. Rest! Conduct only the most necessary of physical activities. Abstain from all food if you have no appetite. With the increased energies, your body will devote itself to a thorough housecleaning and repair measures unlike any you've ever witnessed. Your infirmity is reduced by more than half—healing occurs much faster. At the end, you should feel like new—in fact, you will look greatly rejuvenated because you will be somewhat rejuvenated—recharged for high level function for which we humans are admirably endowed.

All healing power is inherent in the living organism. There is no curative virtue in drugs nor in anything outside the living organism. Nature has not provided remedies for disease. There is no such thing as a "law of cure." The only condition of recovery is obedience to physiological law. So-called remedial agents do not act on the living system, as is taught, but are acted on by the vital organism.

Disease is not, as is commonly supposed, an enemy at war with the powers of the living organism, but is itself a remedial effort—a process of purification and repair. It is not something to be destroyed, subdued, suppressed, killed or cured, but an intelligent body action to be cooperated with. Nature's Materia Hygienica consists of light, air, water, food, temperature, exercise, rest, sleep, abstinence, cleanliness and passional influences.

2.2

SLEEP: THE SOURCE OF YOUR
SELF-HEALING ENERGY

Know your self-healing power! Use the gift of sleep to get well!

The greatest power in the universe is your own life force! The energy that keeps you alive also powers every bit of your healing! Will you use it to your full advantage or ignore and squander it, erroneously assuming your healing power is to be found elsewhere?

Your body is constantly working as best it can to preserve and improve its vital domain: repairing its parts when needed, regenerating, rebalancing and optimizing all of its functions. This healing force is vigorous and thorough, under favorable conditions.

With rare exceptions, your genes contain the perfect instructions for all manner of self-healing; it happens automatically. All that is needed is that we intelligently cooperate with the body's calls for rest so that it can accomplish its tasks without interference. This means stepping out of the way and conserving energy so that our fullest energy potential is available for the healing work.

Our innate body intelligence knows best—it trumps the meddling mind and our futile tinkerings every time! Trust your body's wisdom—let it do its work and your "healing miracle" will take place in its own time. Healing can be fast or slow—we must be patient and accept that the body is always doing its best.

When we are sick or injured, the body's actions are unerring as it goes about its business of restoring health. Occasionally, we may need some form of emergency care and mechanical manipulation to facilitate the natural healing of the entire organism; this should be done in an energy-conserving manner without interfering with the body's self-correcting actions. If we cooperate with the body, providing the optimum conditions for health, the healing job will be accomplished in minimal time.

Squandering our own self-healing power is a tragic mistake made too often by too many. We only delay healing and prolong suffering when we attempt to "fix" or "treat" the body with modalities. The body heals not because of, but in spite of such interventions! Allowing our innate power to do its work, while we patiently ride out the health restoration process, is a beautiful experience; it is always the most prudent approach. Best of all, *it's free!*

Healing is as easy as lying down, closing your eyes and letting the God within take over. Sleep is the most powerful healing remedy! The body is a "self-curing" marvel!

Every day we nearly run out of nerve energy and, as is Nature's way, we fall asleep. This nerve energy is our vitality—it is our most precious commodity, bar none! Nerve energy powers our nervous system, our organs and the self-healing processes and it comes from rest and sleep. *Sleep is the source of our vitality!*

When we are wide awake, the body-mind is active, and nerve energy is being used up—little is available for healing. During sleep, most of our bodily energy is intelligently channeled toward healing. Sleep your way to health and vigorous vitality and feel better soon!

Sleep is your fountainhead of self-healing energy. The more you sleep, the more your vital energy will build up for all of your mind-body functions. Sleep charges your nerve cell "batteries" and fills up your nerve energy "storage tank." It's like "putting money in the bank." When your nerve energy "bank account" is full, you will "feel like a million" and be enabled to heal as quickly as possible! Keep your nerve energy strong via sleep and rest, a simple nutrient-rich rawfood diet and a restful healing program and your body will heal with great vigor!

Sleep and rest are our most productive sources of nerve energy. It does not come from drugs, stimulants such as nutraceuticals and superfoods, "energy drinks" with caffeine, "energy work," therapies or activities of any kind. Rather, they deplete our precious nerve energy through stimulation. Never squander your nerve energy, especially when you are in need of healing, which is all about building up and conserving nerve energy so that the body can use it for the most important tasks at hand. The ultimate healing approach is to take a water fast with bed rest.

Do you feel tired, irritable, cranky, upset or depressed? Is your mind unclear and your ability to reason feeble? Are you healing too slowly or getting nowhere with your health quest? We cannot do anything well when we are short on sleep. Sleep and sleep some more until your energy is restored and you feel renewed— then you will be on your way to vibrant health!

Do you want vigorous energy? Sleep! Do you want to heal? Go to sleep! Do you want to heal faster? Sleep more! Obey your most basic health need and you will be on your way to vibrant health! Remember: you cannot oversleep. Sleep puts "money" in your energy reserve account. Sleep gives you vitality!

You can get something from nothing! Do nothing, intelligently: go to sleep when your body is tired or ailing. When it needs to accomplish extraordinary work, it demands more sleep. The "do nothing" cure is the smartest thing you can do when you need healing. Make it your first, not your last resort! After all, it is free! All else is usually a waste of time, energy and money!

You can spend a fortune going to all the best doctors in the world. Save most of your money and take this million dollar advice: go to sleep and your body will charge up with healing energy and heal. Nothing else can heal you! That's 90% of everything you need to know about healing right there.

Take the sleep challenge, often. There's "nothing" to it and you will marvel at how much better you feel with a "full tank" of nerve energy.

You have the self-healing power! Sleep gives it to us. Call it the "magic elixir of life," the "fountain of youth," "the rejuvenator," "the invigorator," or the "healing miracle worker." It's your personal power plant, your healing sanctuary, the ace up your sleeve, and Nature's great gift!

Always remember: sleep = fastest healing results. That's a direct order from the doctor within!

2.3
UNDERSTANDING DISEASE

by Dr. T. C. Fry and Dr. David Klein

Disease, or "dis-ease," is what we feel when the body is in the process of detoxifying and healing itself. Disease is the body's intelligent response to abnormal or threatening influences. Disease is not something which invades our bodies from outside, nor is it something to be cured or stopped. In a manner of speaking, disease symptoms are a manifestation that the body is "curing" itself.

Disease is instituted by the body itself as an emergency measure to purify and repair itself. Modalities (treatments or therapies that involve drugs, herbs, manipulations or other infringements upon the vital domain) cannot possibly assist the body. On the contrary, they interfere with vital body purification and reparative functions and normal body functions as well. Such interference poses additional problems for the body to cope with, thereby further lowering the body vitality. Body vitality may be lowered so much by the greater danger presented by the drugs or modalities that the original disease effort, which is actually an effort to purify the body, is discontinued in favor of devoting available energies to the more virulent enemy, the drugs within. That is why medical physicians are called "allopaths." That is why there is so much "iatrogenic disease," meaning disease caused by treatments.

"Allopath" literally means "opposite disease." In theory, allopathic doctors strive to displace the original disease by creating a heteropathic or opposite disease. Actually, all physicians succeed in doing is to create additional disease. The original problem remains while the body must redirect its energies partly or wholly to removing the more dangerous drugs, herbs, or so-called medicines. Thus, symptoms of the original disease disappear (or are suppressed and masked) because the necessary energy and vitality to further conduct the disease are now lacking. Yet, the body is in graver danger than before it was treated from both the uneliminated toxic accumulations and the added toxicity of drugs or other substances administered.

The best way to help the body in disease is to "intelligently do nothing" and simultaneously establish conditions of health that enable the body to devote all its vitality to the healing crisis. A thoroughgoing rest under tranquil circumstances constitutes a healing environment, for it permits full devotion of body energies to the emergency task.

The body is always acting intelligently and correctly. The body is always acting appropriately based on the conditions with which it must contend. We can interfere with its operations, but we cannot possibly help it other than by furnishing the normal needs of life consonant with existing body conditions.

In 1926, in his book *Toxemia Explained*, John H. Tilden, M. D., wrote: *"All so-called diseases are merely crises of toxemia and evolve from just one cause: toxemia."* Dr. Tilden further wrote:

"It should be known to all discerning physicians that the earliest stage of organic disease is purely functional, evanescent and never autogenated so far as the affected organ is concerned, but is invariably due to an extraneous irritation (or stimulation, if you please) augmented by toxemia. When the irritation is not continuous and toxin is eliminated as fast as developed to the toleration point, normal functioning is resumed between the intervals of irritation and toxin excess.

"For example: a simple coryza (running at the nose—cold in the head), gastritis or colonitis. At first these colds, catarrhs or inflammations are periodic and functional; but as exciting cause or causes (local irritation and toxemia) becomes more intense and continuous, the mucous membranes of these organs take on organic changes which are given various names such as irritation, inflammation, ulceration and cancer. The pathology (organic change) may be studied until doomsday without throwing any light on the cause, for from the first irritation to the extreme ending—cachexia—which may be given the blanket term "tuberculosis," "syphilis" or "cancer," the whole pathological panorama is one of continuous evolution of intensifying effects."

The *"seven stages of disease"* nominated by Dr. Tilden are: 1. enervation; 2. toxemia, or toxicosis; 3. irritation; 4. inflammation; 5. ulceration; 6. induration; and 7. cancer. It is notable that in some cases even colon cancer has been overcome by making wholistic dietary and lifestyle changes—we obviously want to halt disease at stage one.

By stopping disease symptoms with medicines, a person suffers further toxification and enervation. Disease symptoms may subside with medicines because: 1. the medicine may be so enervating that the body is no longer able to continue with the detoxification process, or 2. the medicine may be so toxic that the body may shift its detoxification efforts to other areas of the body (resulting in new disease symptoms commonly called "side effects").

If a person with inflammatory bowel disease replaces the unhealthful dietary and lifestyle factors which lead to disease with healthful ones, the body will heal itself and ease will be restored.

2.4
HOW AN UNNATURAL DIET CAUSES DISEASES

by Dr. T. C. Fry

Just as kerosene fouls up an automobile or airplane engine which was not designed for it, so, too, will foods foul up human bodies if they are not adapted to them. If you are not physiologically adapted to a diet, it will be repulsive to you in its raw natural state—you cannot relish the food nor sustain yourself on it in good health. When you eat an unnatural diet by artifice, that is, by denaturing it by cooking and modifying and camouflaging its taste with condiments and so on, you are doing the following:

1. Heat-deranging and destroying the nutrients within the food.

2. Deranging your taste buds through excitation with toxic substances to make the unpalatable food acceptable. All poisonous substances impose burdensome eliminative problems upon the body. Sicknesses, ailments and diseases result.

3. Causing nutrient deficiencies by eating a partially or wholly nutrient deranged "food."

4. Causing protein malnutrition. Cooking destroys proteins and amino acids. Once they are oxidized and destroyed by cooking, you can no longer derive any benefit from proteinaceous substances other than, perhaps "empty calories," that is, nutrient-bereft fuel. Once oxidized, proteins are soil (food) for bacteria which putrefy (rot) it. Bacterial putrefactive byproducts are highly toxic and carcinogenic. These byproducts are methane gas (the source for smelly gas emissions when you eat beans, for instance), hydrogen sulfide and mercaptans (which yield the rotten egg smell when carried out by the methane gas), cadaverine, putrescine, ammonias, indoles, skatoles, leukomaines and profusion of other toxic and carcinogenic substances.

5. Laying the groundwork for putrefactive bacterial flora that will vitiate your intestinal tract. Eaters of cooked foods and wrong foods have about two pounds of bacterial flora up and down their digestive tracts. Raw food eaters have only a few ounces.

6. Laying the groundwork for alcohol and vinegar poisoning. Heated sugars and carbohydrates are readily fermented by fungi and bacteria with, first, alcohol as a byproduct and, then, vinegar which is dozens of times more toxic than alcohol.

7. Intoxicating your body with the toxic debris (deranged nutrients) of what once had nutrient value. Instead of materials your body can use, you have toxins that put the body into a frenzy and, if overwhelmed by the toxic load, into a pathological state.

As you can see, cooked foods and condiments (most condiments are toxic plant excitants and stimulants: life-sapping inorganic substances like salt, pathogenic fermentation products like soy sauces, cheeses, etc.) are a curse to our well-being.

There are many toxic substances that are commonly eaten. For instance:

1. Ordinary commercial orange juice contains a carcinogen! Because the whole orange is squeezed, the toxic limonene (a volatile and flammable oil) in the skin is in the juice. The same goes for lemon and grapefruit juices. Refer to the Office of Toxicological Sciences of the Food and Drug Administration (FDA).

2. Ordinary mushrooms contain several toxic substances (mainly hydrazine) that are carcinogenic. This has been reported by researchers at the University of Nebraska Medical School and Dr. Bruce N. Ames of the University of California Biochemistry Department. Refer to the September 23, 1983 issue of Science *magazine.*

3. Tofu, a highly refined soy bean product, contains several carcinogens, notably indole and nitropyrene. Refer to Diet, Nutrition and Cancer.

4. Alfalfa sprouts contain a carcinogen, canavanine. Refer to the September 23, 1983 issue of Science, *and the FDA's Office of Toxicological Sciences.*

5. All cooked and heated oils and fats as in fried foods, nuts, seeds, meats, etc. contain deadly carcinogens. Their aerated fumes are worse in the lungs than tobacco smoke! Refer to Diet, Nutrition and Cancer.

The list seems endless! We Americans poison ourselves so much that we have more health problems per capita than any other country on earth. More than 16% of our national wealth goes down the disease rat hole.

Needless to say, all discomforts, illnesses and suffering are abnormal, unnatural and unnecessary.

2.5
UNDERSTANDING INFLAMMATION

When injured or invaded by toxic matter, gases or microorganisms, or when a buildup of internal toxic debris, fluids and/or microorganisms (commonly called an "infection") reaches a crucial level, the body enacts a health-restorative purification process called inflammation. In this process, the body is working at a "feverish" pace to heal you! It sends elements of the immune system to the threatened area: phagocytes, including monocyte/macrophages and leukocytes, also known as white blood cells or T cells, which produce antibodies, binding toxins to the killer/neutralizing T cells. In the cases of C&C, toxic fecal matter and acid wastes have poisoned the bowel, causing the body to enact inflammation in order to purify the tissues.

In addition to the T cell action, the body sends antibody-producing B cells, more blood and more lymphatic fluid for removal of toxic debris to the threatened area. Also, the permeability of the small blood vessels is increased to permit the delivery of large molecules from the bloodstream to the damaged area for use in the body's repair work. The extra blood and lymphatic fluid causes the inflamed area to swell, redden, feel hot and, sometimes, painful. These are all normal and positive signs of the body's magnificent self-healing powers in action.

Inflammation is vigorous self-healing action intelligently conducted by the body. The intelligence of bodily healing action is supreme, and we must support the process. No matter what we do, only the body can heal itself, and, in each case, it heals in spite of, not because of, our interference. Only the body can heal itself, and there is no force in our lives which is more powerful than its self-healing powers.

If we have internal inflammation, we must remove the causes of disease—ie., toxic diet, drugs, mental/emotional/lifestyle stress, etc.—and supply the body with the conditions of health: clean-digesting nutritious diet, rest, sleep, etc. If the inflammation is external, it is prudent to simply clean the affected area with water, then leave it alone and get plenty of rest and sleep to allow the body to shunt all the self-healing energy it can muster for its restorative job. Inflammation will run its course if we support the self-healing process. Only then will health be restored. Remember: self-healing energy is only generated when we sleep—it does not come from food or remedies or anything else. There are no exceptions to this physiological process of life.

Taking anti-inflammatory medicines and herbs works against the body's restorative action, since all "medicinal" anti-inflammatory agents are toxic and enervating—they have no healing intelligence and do not act on the body; rather, the body works to eliminate them. Thus, their use is counterproductive, decreasing the amount of bodily energy available for self-healing and, in some cases, making us sicker. Overdosing on medicines and herbs can weaken the body so greatly that it has no energy for keeping the inflammation process going, and thus the inflammation stops prematurely, fooling people into believing that the agent "worked." That does not "cure" us; rather, that stops the self-healing action, keeping us toxic! Icing a wound chills out our life-force, slowing down the healing process. The self-healing life-force needs to rage on, unimpeded, to complete its job! And it will, when we provide the conditions of health.

By deeply delving into these simple yet mind-challenging teachings, you will become empowered to heal and live free of fear of disease.

2.6
UNDERSTANDING DETOXIFICATION
AND WEIGHT LOSS

Upon changing to a vibrant, high water content, vegan diet of mostly raw foods, the body begins to improve its state of health, initiating detoxification and health-building actions since it is always striving to establish a higher state of wellness.

The enzymatically-active live raw foods with their nutritious, energizing sugars cause the body to spring into action, utilizing much of its energy in cleaning house: purging debris from the bowels, shedding old inferior cells, and using the new raw nutrients to build a completely new, healthier body. The transition may need to be made gradually to avoid triggering drastic cleansing. However, since most people with C&C are already detoxing at a rapid rate, most can comfortably and safely make a quick transition to the vegan healing diet described herein. You must experiment during the first few days to see what works comfortably for you. As long as there is vitality, the opportunity exists for the body to rejuvenate to a far more vigorous level of health. Results are often noticed within one to three days of beginning this healthful regimen.

Detoxification is a self-purifying process which the body carries out at all times, but most aggressively during the early to late morning hours. It is advantageous to eat lightly in the morning. Heavy foods eaten at this time suspend the cleansing process, keeping us toxic, and, in some cases, overweight. The process of "detox" entails: 1. the cells off-loading metabolic wastes and environmental toxins into the bloodstream for filtering by the liver and kidneys for elimination, and 2. the organs of elimination (bowels, kidneys, lungs, skin, vagina) releasing metabolic, environmental and residual food wastes via feces, urine, breath, sweat and menses. Toxins are also expectorated in mucous via the throat and sinuses.

Under normal conditions of healthful living and natural diet, the body is able to eliminate metabolic wastes and other environmental pollutants through its normal organs of elimination. However, under chronic excessive bombardment with unnatural dietary fare, environmental pollutants, emotional stress, and/or over-eating (of even good natural foods), the body's eliminative capacities are not equal to the task. A buildup of toxins increases as the days and years go by, especially in the bowels. This condition, called toxicosis, leads to accelerated aging, fatigue, illness, and, in many cases, obesity. In this condition of toxicity, which is particularly likely if one has lived on a diet of foods such as cooked meat, dairy, bread, and junk foods, the body harbors sticky and insoluble debris and waste matter in the bowels, on artery walls and in the bloodstream, tissues and other organs.

Fortunately, the body is a magnificently designed masterpiece of self-healing, always striving to establish and maintain purity and wellness. When a toxic load becomes too dangerous for the body, it intelligently enacts a detoxification/elimination event or phase, manifested by any of these "symptoms": sore throat, inflammation, fever, skin outbreaks, coated tongue, mucous expectoration, body aches, nausea, vomiting and diarrhea. Malodorous body wastes and underarms are signs that toxic, putrid, fermented matter and acids are being eliminated. During the detoxification phase, many people experience lightheadedness and headaches as the body stirs up and dumps toxins into the bloodstream for processing and elimination. During a thorough detox, unhealthy fat, cysts and even tumors are also broken down (autolyzed) and eliminated. As toxins are stirred up and released, the body relaxes and people also typically experience short-term symptoms of mental-emotional detoxification: mood swings, depression, sadness, anger and crying.

With this process, everyone also experiences weight loss, which is absolutely necessary as the body rids itself of toxic, morbid food matter stored in the bowels and tissues, unhealthy fat and other toxins in order to restore health and rebuild itself with all new healthy cells. A clean internal environment is essential for this healing and rejuvenation work. As such, weight loss must be welcomed and not feared. The body will not lose anything it needs; the poison must come out. The body knows exactly what it is doing during the detox; we must cooperate and allow it to clean out the threatening matter. When properly implemented, the healing program taught herein is safe and results in superior nutrification and health. Healthy weight and robust energy will gradually be gained after healing is complete and medicines are discontinued. There are no shortcuts to health; after C&C we must totally clean out, establish a clean inner environment and maintain the healthful lifestyle practices for the duration of our lives. If we do not clean out or maintain inner cleanliness, C&C will return.

Detox is often initially unpleasant, but as "dis-ease" symptoms diminish it becomes a dramatically wonderful process as you know you are healing. When the organs of elimination are weak and/or overloaded, the body will resort to eliminating toxins through any convenient outlet it can find, e.g., the eyes, ears, throat, vagina, skin (sweating, rashes, fissures and suppurations), sinuses and scalp. When we experience any of these signs of elimination, we typically feel fatigued and sleepy, as the body is directing much of its energy toward accomplishing the housecleaning. At such times, it is always wise to assist the body by heeding the calls for extra rest and sleep. All of these "symptoms" will lessen and then vanish when the body is sufficiently cleaned out, providing we adhere to a healthful lifestyle regimen.

In conjunction with the heightened detoxification action, the body works at repairing any damage, regenerating new cells, rejuvenating and restoring wellness. The repair work mostly occurs when we sleep. When there is damage to be repaired and rejuvenation to be accomplished, the body needs extra sleep. We typically feel weak and need plenty of extra sleep in the beginning stage of the rejuvenation phase. If the toxemia, physical damage, degeneration and emotional distress are severe, this phase may last for weeks or months. It is important to understand that the symptoms of the detoxification and healing process signify the workings of the awesome rejuvenative power of the body. It will help the process if we appreciate the workings of the body and do everything possible to assist it in its healing processes. We can do this by taking a break or a sabbatical from our normal routines, obtaining plenty of extra sleep and rest—if necessary, complete rest—as well as eating simply until the work is sufficiently accomplished and we experience new vigor and vitality. It would be ideal to take the sabbatical at a comfortable health center or retreat with fasting supervision (if needed), juicing, deep rest and Natural Hygiene education.

If we persevere through the uncomfortable detoxification symptoms, including the concomitant weight loss, and stick with the healing and healthful lifestyle program, getting extra sleep and rest when feeling tired or unwell, and resisting covering up symptoms with medicines (which only add more toxins to the system), we will arrive at a wonderful state of well-being in the quickest time possible, gain new healthy weight and stronger muscles, and, in the process, we will learn invaluable lessons about how the body works to restore health. Generally, two to six months are needed for the body to accomplish its grand healing work and begin healthy weight gain. There are no shortcuts to health; we must cooperate with the body's needs and be patient. Some of the rewards for sticking with this health program include freedom from illness (no more flare-ups!), sweet-smelling breath, no body odors, easy and inoffensive elimination, shinier, thicker hair, clearer eyes and skin, more mental energy and clarity, better memory, more joie de vivre, slimmer belly, no cellulite, greater physical strength and stamina, deeper connection to spirit, finding a mutual attraction with healthy, vivacious people like ourselves and superior longevity. Through healthful living practices which keep our bodies clean inside and free of energy-robbing toxic matter, we can ensure a healthier, longer, more vital and youthful life, free ourselves from disease and aging and tap into the wellspring of joy within. Welcome the detox and give your body the thorough rest it is demanding!

2.7
NATURAL HYGIENE: THE SCIENCE AND FINE ART OF HEALTHFUL LIVING

by Dr. T. C. Fry and Dr. David Klein

Natural Hygiene, or Healthful Living, is the art and science of living healthfully in accord with our natural biological heritage. Natural Hygiene embodies those principles which guide us to correct living practices. It is a health system of cooperating with Nature to allow our self-healing powers to fully express themselves, enabling the body to rejuvenate and establish its highest level of health. "Hygiene" literally means "the science of health."

Natural Hygiene is about enhancing physical, emotional, mental and spiritual well-being through education and right living. It provides us with a simple, wholistic, living awareness system for regaining and maintaining superb human health and beauty. Hygiene is personally empowering and liberating. It teaches independence and rational action. It banishes fear and ignorance regarding human health and how to keep it. Ultimately, it is about freedom.

Natural Hygiene always refers to nature as its mentor and teacher. When wholistic, comprehensive understanding is required, one must refer back to nature in its pristine majesty as the final authority. Because present-day life seems to be losing touch with those conditions which made life possible, Natural Hygiene brings us "back to the garden," so to speak. We should strive to meet life's requirements, and to smoothly balance them in all aspects so that we can easily lead a joyous and fulfilling existence.

Natural Hygiene concerns itself with those principles and truths applicable to human life so that we may wisely apply them to our lives. We are of the firm conviction that only by living healthfully can we realize the loftiest joys, peace of mind and blissful connection with all of creation which is our birthright.

Animals in nature are creatures of instinct. Following the guidance of instinct, they are correctly self-directed to meet their needs. They thrive optimally in accord with their environmental and genetic possibilities. Discovering and attuning to our natural instincts is part and parcel of Natural Hygiene. Our inborn guiding instincts always tend toward healthful and constructive living when they are unclouded and given proper attention. It is ignorance of our instincts and the laws of life that creates our sickness and suffering.

In presenting the concept that health is normal and natural, Natural Hygienists emphatically refute the idea that disease is inevitable in our lives. We contend that disease will not occur unless there is sufficient cause. Health maintenance is an unceasing process in every organism. When the organism is overwhelmed by toxic substances beyond its ability to eliminate them in normal course, the body institutes emergency action to effect expulsion of the toxic burden. This crisis is called "sickness" or "disease." Toxic materials accumulate in the body from two sources: 1. from unexpelled body wastes that are endogenously generated as a normal part of our metabolism, and 2. from exogenous materials ingested and partially or wholly retained due to inability to cope with the eliminative load.

All the needs of normal physiology are present in states of disease and are required to be supplied to the end that organic and functional integrity may be preserved or restored. No piecemeal plan of care can possibly succeed in restoring health. Hygienic care comprehends not only a regulation of the diet, but a synthesis and coordination of all the factor elements of normal living: drinking, breathing, sunning, temperature, clothing, exercise, rest, sleep, emotional factors, etc. Nothing short of a total regulation of the way of life can produce ideal results.

All processes of recovery or healing are but extensions and modifications of the processes that preserve health. The materials and processes employed in caring for the sick must be in consonance with physiology and compatible with all other useful measures. A sane method of caring for the sick will not force the body to utilize substances that are not subject to its metabolic processes.

Our biological nature, i.e., the make-up (structure, function and living essence) of our bodies, determines our needs and how we should meet them. Health is our natural state of being. Disease processes (or illnesses) are perfectly natural responses enacted by the body for the purpose of detoxifying, rebalancing, adapting to harmful influences and healing. The condition of health (or wellness) is only achieved by living healthfully, i.e., satisfying our mental/emotional/physiological/spiritual needs.

The Hygienic health system of self-healing has a 200-year track record, establishing it as the most effective healing system ever known to man. The true Hygienic art consists of applying to the living system whatever materials and conditions it can use under the circumstances, and not in the administration of poisons which it must resist and expel. Drugs are themselves causes of disease and produce disease whenever given. They cure nothing. The drug system endeavors to make the sick well by administering poisons which make well persons sick.

Natural Hygiene, on the contrary, restores the sick to health by the means that preserve health in well persons. Disease is caused by violations of the laws and conditions of life. The Hygienic System stops the violations and supplies healthful conditions. Drug medication adds to the causes of destruction and metamorphoses acutely into chronic disease where it does not kill outright. The attempt to cure disease by adding to its causes is irrational and absurd. Hygienic care involves the proper use of all Hygienic materials and influences of nature but rejects all poisons. There is, therefore, between the Hygienic System and the Drug System an irrepressible con-

flict. If one is true, the other is false.

We must eliminate the dead weight of false knowledge and ideas that we carry with us each moment. Using treatments, drugs, herbs, or anything else abnormal and unnatural to the body can interfere with healthful body functions but, under no circumstances, can these agencies heal the body. Because these devitalizing agencies depress and suppress symptoms (or evidences) of body healing efforts, and because the body discontinues vital activities to contend with these agencies, which makes the symptoms disappear, the anti-vital effects of drugs and treatments are mistaken for healing effects. Nothing but the body can heal itself.

2.8
THE HEALTHFUL LIVING CREDO OF LIFE

by Dr. T. C. Fry

Attuning to our natural instincts and aligning with Nature is part and parcel of Healthful Living. We are of the firm conviction that only by living healthfully can we realize the loftiest joys and destiny which are our birthright. Two centuries of unfailing results have proven Healthful Living, which is synonymous with Natural Hygiene, to be the true science of health and the greatest healthful living practice humanity has ever known.

Healthful Living holds that life should be meaningful and filled with beauty, love, kindness, goodness and happiness.

Healthful Living holds that we are naturally good, righteous, loving, sharing and virtuous, and that our exalted character will manifest under ideal life conditions.

Healthful Living holds that superlative well-being is normal to our existence and is necessary to the achievement of our highest potential.

Healthful Living holds that supreme human excellence can be realized only in those who embrace those precepts and practices which are productive of superb well-being.

Healthful Living, which encompasses all that bears upon human well-being, and which bases itself soundly upon the human biological and spiritual heritage, constitutes the way to realize the highest possible order of human existence.

Healthful Living is in harmony with nature, in accord with the principles of vital organic existence, correct in science, sound in philosophy, ethics, environment, economics, and animal rights, agreement with common sense, successful in practice and a blessing to humankind.

Healthful Living recognizes that the human body is self-constructing, having developed from a fertilized ovum, that it is self-preserving, that it is self-defending and, through the mighty power and intelligence that constructed it, totally self-cleansing and self-repairing.

Healthful Living recognizes that the body maintains itself in perfect health, completely free of disease, if its needs are correctly met.

Healthful Living recognizes that humans are biologically and anatomically frugivores and are constitutionally, anatomically and aesthetically adapted to a diet primarily of fruits and, secondarily, nuts, seeds and vegetables. Ideally, they must be eaten in the fresh, raw, natural state in combinations that are compatible in digestive chemistry.

Healthful Living recognizes that diseases are caused by the body in response to improper life practices, especially dietary indiscretions. Illness proceeds from reduced nerve energy and consequent toxicosis from internally generated wastes, from ingested substances bearing or begetting toxicity, or from a combination of both. Insufficient nerve energy arises from dissipation, stress, overindulgence, excess or deficiency of the normal essentials of life, or not normal to it. Accordingly, recovery from sickness can be achieved only by removing the causes and establishing conditions favorable to recovery.

Healthful Living recognizes that a thoroughgoing rest, which includes fasting (physical, emotional, sensory, and physiologic rest), is the most favorable condition under which an ailing body can purify and restore itself.

Healthful Living, which teaches that exalted well-being can be attained and maintained only through biologically correct living practices, is not in any sense a healing art or a curing cult. It regards as mistaken and productive of much grief the idea that disease can be prevented or overcome by agencies abnormal to our natural being. Consequently, Healthful Living emphatically rejects drugs, medications, vaccinations and treatments because they undermine health by suppressing, disrupting or destroying vital body processes, functions, cells and tissues.

Therefore, Healthful Living regards body and mind as the inviolable sanctuary of an individual's being. Healthful Living holds that everyone has an inalienable right to have a pure and uncontaminated body, to be free of abnormal compulsions and restraints, and to be free to meet his or her needs as a responsible member of society.

2.9
THE PRIME REQUISITES OF HEALTH

1. Love of Self
2. Healthy Self-image and Esteem
3. Passionate Love of All Life
4. Awareness
5. Intention
6. Inner Focus/Listening
7. Abidance by the Senses and Intuition
8. True Knowledge
9. Graceful, Grateful, Respectful, Generous Attitude
10. Organic, Properly-combined Vegan Diet
11. Pure Water
12. Pure Air
13. Sunshine
14. Warm Climate
15. Fitness and Posture
16. Security and Peace of Mind
17. Rejuvenative Rest and Sleep
18. Heart-centered Self Nurturing
19. Sharing of Love
20. Relaxation
21. Humor
22. Creative Expression
23. Emotional Flow and Release
24. Rhythmic Movement
25. Musical Indulgence
26. Simple Lifestyle
27. Communing With Nature
28. Gardening
29. Service—Living Your Life's Purpose
30. Engagement in Self-improvement Challenges

By living hygienically, or healthfully, we are enabled to rejuvenate and reach our full health potential.

2.10
CORRECT WAYS OF LIVING ARE ESSENTIAL!

by Dr. T. C. Fry

If we demand a correction of the ways of life as the one and only means of securing a restoration of health, we will be patronized by the millions who still believe that among the myriad of so-called cures there is palliation (reduction of symptoms) for them and are content with only palliation. There is a mighty army of invalids today who cannot get well in spite of their travels, their patronage of the great specialists and their submission to operations, but they are still unwilling to make a few simple corrections in their ways of living in the interest of better health.

When one of these sufferers does condescend to break away from the cures of science and to undertake a wholly new and, to him or her, untried way back to health, he or she is often in a desperate condition. Much organic derangement has occurred so that nothing short of the creation of a new organ can restore full health. We don't expect such sufferers to recover full health, but we do witness some remarkable improvements in great numbers of these desperate cases. In the less damaged, we see great numbers of full recoveries.

2.11
WHAT IT TAKES TO GET WELL

by Dr. Herbert M. Shelton

You have tried drugs and treatments for months or years. These have all failed you. Your health has steadily deteriorated under such direction. You have reached the end of your faith and confidence in these modalities. You are ready to try something else; perhaps you are grasping at straws. Glowing accounts of restoration of health under Hygienic care have reached you. You have heard that the lame, halt, blind, deaf, bedridden and well-nigh dead have been restored to good health—have risen, as by the touch of magic, to full, bounding, rosy-cheeked health. And you long to matriculate, to have your name enrolled in a Hygienic institution.

Hygienic Measures Can Restore Health

Now, Hygiene is worthy of your highest consideration. It has demonstrated its efficacy to the amplest satisfaction of its friends and devotees. It has more than met their expectations. But it will not do for you to judge it in the light of reports of magic renovations, which are exceptional. They constitute no safe basis for judgment, and when relied on serve only to disappoint, for facts are otherwise, and nothing is gained by deception or misrepresentation.

The vast number of those who turn to Hygiene in their search for health are very sick persons. Hygiene has always relied on the operations of the forces of the organism, and these forces know nothing of magic. For good or ill, and as a general rule, they change bodily structures slowly. Assuming that you have long been sick, and that you have been so much tampered with by drugs, the integrity of the powers of your life have been seriously reduced and perverted. Your instincts and reduced powers have made you somewhat feeble and impaired your abilities to do what you normally could. What may you reasonably expect to result from an adaptation of the means of Hygiene? How far can you expect to have your weakened organs strengthened, your damaged structures repaired, your impaired functions restored, your sluggish circulation invigorated and your lowered powers recuperated?

Body Reinvigoration is Not a Fast Process

If you entertain the idea that all of this can be done in a few days or even a few weeks, it is not a reasonable expectation. A week or two of rest and fasting, a short time on a vastly improved diet, a correction of the habits of life—these cannot be expected to perform miracles. It is necessary to disabuse your mind of the thought that the wreckage of years of wrong living can be cleared away and your weakened and impaired organism renewed and refurbished in short order. Hygienists claim for Hygiene no such magic virtues. They never did. In this, Hygiene has been misrepresented by overly enthusiastic and ill-informed friends.

There is No Miraculous Way to Health

What Hygiene does claim is far different from all this. What it does claim is that where recovery is still possible, by means of Hygienic measures and materials, health can be restored more rapidly, more safely, more efficiently and more certainly than when these means are neglected. It does not claim to cure disease; it does not claim to be able to reverse irreversible pathologies; it does not claim that health can be restored instantly. It knows nothing of hocus-pocus, has no incantations, adopts no mummeries, attempts no cheateries, avoids the pretensions of the empiric, the loud noise of the charlatan and the abracadabra of the drug-giver.

Hygiene makes full use of the life-sustaining and health-giving means of nature—placing its full reliance on those means that have a natural relation to physiology—and depends upon the restorative forces intrinsic to the organism to do the actual work of repair and reconstruction. If this is quackery, then life is a quack and nature one grand cheat.

Health Depends on Meeting Body Needs

Hygienic plans, processes and means are, so far as they go, transcripts of the laws of nature, as expressed in the realm of biology. The food it employs, the exercise it requires, the rest it enforces, the sunshine it makes use of, the abstinence required, the corrections of the ways of life it requires are all employed with special relations to the physiological requirements of the body and not with relation to some supposed need to cure disease. The human organism and its needs, the laws of its actions and reactions, govern the employment of Hygienic means. To fully understand the principles and parts of the steam engine enable us to know what is essential to maintain it in order. To know what will keep it in order is to know what is necessary to put it in order when it is out of order. So it is with the human constitution. To know the means whose legitimate uses keep the body in health is also to know the means that are necessary to restore health. To restore health, exactly those same means are required, though it may be in different measure which, were one well, would tend—naturally and normally—to keep one well. Thus, when we know what are the means of keeping people well, we know what will enable them to get well if health is no longer possible.

Health is Normal

The sick always recover when they do by, or through, or in harmony with, the laws which govern their being. Now, it is a fact that change of structure or function or condition from health to sickness is slow. Rarely does one become sick suddenly.

Preparative processes are long at work; underminings proceed for weeks, months, even years, before sickness becomes evident, for the essential condition of life is health. As surely as man is constituted to live, so is he constituted for health. Sickness is an interloper, not a normal state of the living organism. It is the result of long-indulged causes that are foreign to the normal activities of life.

Disease Comes Slowly

Great wastes of energy or profuse expenditures of the powers of the body are needful to the evolution of disease. This being true, can it reasonably be supposed that changes from sickness to health can be rapid? Surely this cannot be so, for if the powers of the organism which are necessary to preserve health have become diminished so that disease has resulted, they must operate feebly in the restoration of health, even under the best of circumstances. The greater the debility, the longer the violations of life's laws, and the more impaired the structures and functions of life, the slower must be the process of recovery.

Under such conditions, the forces of reconstruction and recuperation work at great odds. Their effects in the direction of renewal and repair accumulate little by little. The time required to restore health should not be as long as the time required to get sick, for in getting sick one works against the normal tendencies and health-ward operations of the body, while in getting well, one works with the forces of nature. But one cannot expect to repair the damages produced by years of wrong living in a short time. Play fair with yourself; give yourself a chance. Don't expect miracles for there are none.

We're Blessed With Numerous Guardian Angels

In getting sick, you have been compelled to overcome hosts of "guardian angels" that are integral to your body. Before the causes of disease could tear down your own beautiful structures, these normal safeguards of life had to be overpowered. When wrong living has won a victory over life's normal safeguards, it has nearly wrought our organic ruin. You, to be more specific, by your unwise use of substances contrary to the human disposition and by a thousand other follies, have brought about your own suffering.

We Cause Our Own Suffering

Yet, having brought about the wreckage of a splendid and powerful organism, you talk and act as though Hygiene, to be good for anything worthy of your or others' confidence, should be able to quickly rebuild your ruined constitution—perhaps to better than its original beauty— somewhat on the order of the rearing of the palaces built by the possessor of Aladdin's lamp. Natural processes do not work this way. For you there is no exemption from the lawful and orderly processes of life; there is no royal road to redemption; there is no forgiveness in nature.

Long-continued violation of the laws of being is the cause of disease. Long-continued perseverance in obedience is the only means by which health can be recovered. If the inherent recuperative power is unable to cope with the impairment under conditions of obedience, we may be sure that it will be still less able to cope with both the impairment and the poisons of the physician that may be used to treat the disease. Violated law can never be compensated for by the use of drugs and artificial means. Vitality can be reduced to the extent that symptoms disappear, but wellness is further away than ever.

Healing Takes Place
Only If We Observe the Needs of Life

If healing ever takes place in your wrecked body, it will be in reward for your unwearied patience and perseverance in adhering to a physiologically legitimate way of life. You will have to work. You will have to meet the requirements of life. Steady and persistent obedience to the laws of being, made cheerful and pleasant by a strong confidence in the uniform processes of nature, will bring you back to whatever degree of health, as represented by restored structural integrity and functional vigor, of which you may still be capable.

Man should be taught that health is the normal state and that disease is abnormal. He should be made to understand that he is proof against attack by germs, viruses, fungi and parasites until his normal health has become depressed by enervating habits which inhibit secretion and excretion. Checked elimination results in the accumulation in the body of matabolin, or metabolic waste—a normal (but toxic) byproduct of physiological activities; this is to say, of the processes of life. Man is poised between health and disease, with both the conservative and destructive powers within his control.

Disease is Not Inevitable

To inculcate in every mind that comes into the world the fallacy that disease is inescapable is to make of every human being an easy victim of the high-powered salesmen who traffic in the cure of the various curing systems. All the so-called schools of medicine are very busy impressing on the minds of the people the fear that they will suffer with disease, and that to escape, their cures are needed. With an array of instruments of precision and a variety of clever laboratory techniques, they easily demonstrate to the complete satisfaction of their intended victims that they're victims of maladies requiring expert skills to eradicate.

The Medical Cartel Thrives on
Ignorance and Misconception

The teaching is that man is a victim of entities—germs, viruses, fungi and parasites—that enter the body and against which man has either no natural or normal defenses or weak ones. The cure-mongers, the treatment peddlers, go charging through human tissues in hot pursuit of these evil entities in their efforts to save lives. They work on the theory that the entity can be attacked at its work and its influence rendered negligible, either by some immunization scheme or by some of their many cures.

Knowledge Frees Us of Error

Humans must learn that health is a result of obedience to the laws of life that are as unchangeable as the law of gravity; disease is the result of violations of the same laws. Health is to be restored by a return to obedience of organic law. To imagine that we can restore health while continuing to violate the laws of organic being is tantamount to thinking that these laws are without force, that they can be nullified and set aside at will.

The Laws of Life are Violated in Two Ways:

1. By misusing things which are normally needed by the living organism in its normal activities and developments.

2. By attempting to use things which are abnormal to the organism.

The Elements of Health

Hygienic materials, influences and conditions are only those which are involved in and are essential to the normal operations, developments and activities of life. They are such things and conditions, and those only, as are normally related to the living organism. Such things and conditions as natural food, air, water, sunshine, warmth, exercise, rest and sleep, cleanliness, emotional poise, etc. constitute the ample Materia Hygienica. Except for surgery in certain types of abnormalities, Hygienic substances and conditions are all that can be helpful to the sick organism.

Disease is a Body-Cleansing and Healing Process

A fundamental error of all the schools of so-called medicine has been the assumption that disease is something at war with life and that it must be met, subdued, counteracted, cast out, killed or cured with substances that are antagonistic to the body itself. They have never adequately recognized the antagonism that exists between the living organism and the chemical substances with which they seek to cure disease. This is the reason they continue to fill the bodies of the sick with poisons (foreign or non-usable chemicals) which the body must resist and expel. Not only have such causes of disease been mistaken as remedies for disease, but in some cases they have been mistaken for food.

A knowledge of the vital laws, the special laws of organic nature as distinct from chemical and mechanical laws, will result in the reversal of this practice. Such knowledge will enable people to understand that the best way to care for the sick is to remove the causes of sickness and not to suppress the vital struggle against impurities or poisons. It would teach them to provide the body with what it needs and can use rather than try to force upon it things that it cannot use, does not need, and will have to expel.

All Drugs Impair and Disturb Body Functions— Physicians Can Be Dangerous to Your Well-Being

The introduction of elements into the body that are unadaptable to the normal metabolic processes cannot result in anything but disturbance and impairment of function. By what conceivable means can they enhance the precise and adequate processes of life? How can they have the power and intelligence to further restorative efforts? There is no doubt that the administration of a poison will necessitate a change of activity on the part of the body; that it may temporarily be forced to cease or reduce its work of freeing itself of the causes of disease, while it redirects its attentions and cleansing powers to the drug.

Those symptoms that constitute cellular and organic activities in keeping the body clean may cease for the time being and not again be resumed until the body has expelled the much more dangerous drug. Drugs are, therefore, destructive of the powers of life.

The Body Always Tries to Maintain Normalcy

Those abnormal actions of the body—nausea, vomiting, diarrhea, coughing, sneezing, frequent urination, skin eruptions, fever, pain, vertigo, inflammation, expectoration, prostration, etc.—which we call disease, are the body's remedial struggles. They represent the efforts of the organism to expel injurious substances and to recover the normal state. Such remedial efforts should not be suppressed (with "cures") or interfered with by minuscule intellects. Instead, they should be cooperated with. Instead of quelling the cough, suppressing the diarrhea, reducing the fever, silencing the pain, etc., we should seek to remove the causes that have made these remedial efforts necessary and to supply such Hygienic conditions and materials that the laboring organism can make constructive use of, to the end that it may carry forward its remedial work, that is the restoration of vibrant health, to a successful completion.

It is notorious that the credulity of the people, as related to health and disease and their faith in pills, potions, and wonder drugs as means of restoration of health, is in direct proportion to the ignorance of their own bodies and the true causes of disease. So long as this ignorance persists, there will be plenty of disease-treaters who will take advantage of it and pander to the demand for relief from symptoms.

The Miraculous Powers of the Living Organism

Living beings are fully self-sufficient entities with inherent faculties for main-

taining a state of vigorous well-being if needs are properly supplied and if injurious factors and influences are not indulged in or allowed. The body always strives for a state of internal balance: it creates and maintains an internal environment that conduces to the highest level of function. Upon this equilibrium is based its operating systems. This homeostasis is necessary for optimum function and well-being.

Intelligence and wisdom of an unimaginably high order are involved in maintaining body integrity with such accurate balance. With such a narrow margin of invariability, even laboratories find it difficult to establish and maintain such accurate controls upon physical and chemical substances.

The body at all times maintains, preserves and defends itself. If injured, it immediately begins processes of repair to restore high operational vigor. The body was endowed with an unerring and reliable lifetime repair kit.

Repeat: Only an intelligence of an incredibly high order can operate and maintain such a marvelous system as the human body exhibits. This innate operating intelligence and wisdom dwarf all the knowledge and wisdom of our greatest geniuses.

All Powers of Life Are Within the Organism

Any effort to control the body function amounts to abnormal interference, and all interference is injurious to the body. All powers of life are within the body, and all the accumulated knowledge in the world has yet to improve a single one of these powers. Much has been done to injure and destroy these powers. All efforts to help the body with treatments and so-called healing substances merely interfere with and impede health restoration by giving the body additional burdens with which to contend.

The highest powers of the body are maintained only if the elements on which it thrives optimally are supplied to it. Just as an auto runs great on the finest gasoline for which it was designed and will become sluggish and grind to a halt on kerosene, so, too, the body will operate at its highest possible level on the finest foods and influences to which it was, in its millions of years of development, carefully adapted.

We Are Our Own Worst Enemies

Just as the finest practices, foods and life influences build and maintain life on the highest possible level, so, too, poor and faulty living practices, second-rate and third-rate foods and life-sapping influences lower this level of well-being, impair the organism and destroy it long before its time.

Just as a watch will last many years if kept clean and in fine operating condition—and will keep poor time and quickly become ruined if dust, dirt, etc., are permitted free entry—so, too, it is with the human body. Give the human body only those elements to which it is ideally adapted and it will give only pleasure and joys to its occupant. Give it junk foods, drugs and poor practices and it becomes clogged *up and impaired—it becomes diseased. Its functions are disrupted. Its needs are not properly met so that it can maintain normal high function. Faulty living practices and junk foods cripple the organism so that suffering ensues. This suffering takes the form of sickness or disease. Disease is a form of body crisis—a healing crisis.*

Disease is a Body Emergency Action and is Beneficial

If through poor living practices the body becomes intolerably toxic, the body's vital powers institute an emergency cleansing crisis. It deprives us of discretionary energies. It redirects these energies to the extraordinary task of healing, that is, the processes of cleansing itself of toxic matters and repairing any damage which may have been suffered. To try to "cure" the disease is a laughably ignorant attempt. Disease is a body-healing crisis, and to interfere with it is to impair the processes. To so poison and treat the system with drugs and herbs so that its vital powers must be diverted from the healing processes to the removal of newly introduced toxic matters—drugs injected or ingested that are even more damaging to the vital domain—is sheer lunacy if done innocently, and criminal if done knowingly. Yet, these damaging practices characterize those inflicted upon humanity by the brightest minds of so-called "medical science," which is neither medicine nor science.

If we so live as to bring our bodies to a low state so that it goes into an emergency crisis of elimination, that is, if it disables itself and starts cleansing and repair actions we call colds, inflammations (itises), etc., we'd best cooperate by ceasing eating and all activities. Bed rest in an airy, sunlit room with pure water permits the body full application of its powers to restorative processes. Treating and drugging the body so that it can no longer exercise these vital powers will make the symptoms go away—but this gives rise to even more serious problems down road, whether we realize it or not.

Chronic diseases result from body interference with healing crises. In fact, most degenerative diseases such as cancer, diabetes, heart disease, mental aberrations, etc. result from continued treatments and drugs as much as from continued indulgence of the initial causes. It's like trying to put out a fire with gasoline!

Body Intelligence Reigns Supreme

We must respect our body intelligence. It is greater than all the accumulated knowledge of humankind. Certainly the institutionalized ignorance of so-called medical science has not one answer for human well-being. If a person is drowning, its answer seems to be to try to sink the body instead of rescue it by letting body intelligence take over completely.

There are no secrets in nature! There is only human ignorance. Any attempt to try to improve upon something that needs no improving is injurious and will further degrade the lot of humans. Our degradation begins with the practices that bring on the first cold of infancy and is aggravated by the treatments that then begin. Diseases will not occur unless we cause them. The only way not to cause them is to live in accordance with the laws or biological principles of human life.

Perfect Health Comes From Healthful Practices

Natural Hygiene teaches that to have perfect health, we must adopt a program that will build and maintain perfect health. It teaches that we must abjure injurious practices and habits. We certainly must not indulge in poisonous habits that supply nothing the body needs but give it multitudinous problems with which to contend.

The most salient and offensive of these habits is indulging in tobaccos, coffees, alcohols, teas, chocolates, vinegars, drugs, medicines, etc. And, of course, we must not overlook the junk foods that damage rather than sustain the body, notably: fried foods; cooked foods; milk and milk products, especially cheese and ice cream; candy; flavored, sweetened and drugged drinks; pizzas and other highly condimented concoctions; pastries, cakes, pies and breads; meats and other animal products; fermented and rotted products, such as cheese, sauerkraut, pickles, etc.; and a whole long list of other harmful substances ingested for "kicks" and as foods.

Study Natural Hygiene books if you want to learn what to do to realize vibrant, sickness-free well-being.

2.12
THE LAWS OF LIFE

The Laws of Life were elaborated by the great Natural Hygiene pioneers, Sylvester Graham (1794-1851) and Robert Walter, M.D. (1861-1921). They describe the physiological laws which govern bodily functions with regard to the cause and effect of external influences and its mechanisms of self-preservation and wellness. They serve as the physiological basis for health science (Natural Hygiene) and must be understood by everyone, especially doctors.

We must study and learn to abide by these laws while casting away conventional, contrary errant beliefs which undermine our ability to heal and manifest wellness. In defying the Laws, we fall into the perilous trap of fooling ourselves with stimulants, treatments and therapies which only serve to shift symptoms while robbing us of energy and prolonging our suffering. In understanding and abiding by the Laws, we are empowered to utilize our God-given self-healing power to its fullest extent and manifest the healthy life of our loftiest dreams.

Below is a brief summary of the Laws of Life. An in-depth discussion is beyond the scope of this book. For further study, read books on the subject of Natural Hygiene by Dr. Herbert M. Shelton and others.

1. **Life's Great Law:** *Every particle of living matter in the organized body is endowed with an instinct of self-preservation, sustained by a force inherent in the organism, usually called "vital force" or "life," the success of which is directly proportional to the amount of the force and, inversely, to the degree of activity.*

2. **The Law of Action:** *Whenever action occurs in the living organism as the result of extraneous influences, the action must be ascribed to the living thing, which has the power of action, and not to the dead, whose leading characteristic is inertia.*

3. **The Law of Power:** *The power employed, and, consequently, expended in any vital or medicinal action is vital power, that is, power from within.*

4. **The Law of Selective Elimination:** *All injurious substances which, by any means, gain admittance into the domain of vitality are counteracted, neutralized, and eliminated in such a manner and through such channels as will produce the least amount of wear and tear to the organism.*

5. **The Law of Dual Effect:** *The secondary effect upon the living organism of any act, habit, indulgence, or agent is the exact opposite and equal of the primary effect.*

6. **The Law of Special Economy:** *The vital organism, under favorable conditions, stores up all excess of vital funds above the current expenditure as a reserve*

fund to be employed in a time of special need.

7. The Law of Vital Distribution: *In proportion to the importance and need of the various organs and tissues of the body is the power of the body, whether much or little, apportioned out among them.*

8. The Law of Limitation: *Whenever and wherever the expenditure of vital power has advanced so far that a fatal exhaustion is imminent, a check is put upon the unnecessary expenditure of power and the organism rebels against the further use of even an accustomed "stimulant."*

9. The Law of Vital Accommodation—Nature's Balance Wheel: *The response of the vital organism to external stimuli is an instinctive one, based upon a self-preserving instinct which adapts itself to whatever influence it cannot destroy or control.*

3
THE COLON

3.1
FUNCTIONS OF THE BOWEL

The bowel, also referred to as the intestines or gut, consists of the small and large intestines (the latter is also known as the colon). Here are the basic functions of each:

Small Intestine

The small intestine is a muscular 21-foot long tube of small diameter (about one inch, hence the name "small" intestine). This is where the digestive process takes place. Macronutrients are reduced to sugars, amino acids and fatty acids, then absorbed, along with some micronutrients, and transported to the liver, then distributed to the cells through the blood and lymph. The pH in a healthy small intestine is alkaline.

More specifically, here is what happens during the digestive process. From the stomach, the small intestine receives a semi-digested mixture of food and acidic enzymes; this mixture is called "chyme." The small intestine also receives pancreatic enzyme from the pancreas and bile (a fat emulsifier) from the gall bladder. While being transported through the small intestine by segmentation movement, the digested fluid mass is absorbed through the striated border epithelium covering the villi (the intricate, microscopic finger-like folds which number in the millions).

The bacteria which live on living vegetable foods produce digestive enzymes which assist in the body's digestion of vegetable foods. Under various conditions of poor, haphazard eating and incomplete digestion, however, bacterial decomposition of food occurs (fermentation and putrefaction), resulting in toxic byproducts which can be responsible for irritation, then inflammation, of the intestinal wall. These toxins are typically absorbed into the bloodstream, causing fatigue and a host of illness symptoms. When the wall of the small intestine is inflamed, the nerves and absorptive function of this organ become greatly impaired, and the act of eating is usually met with severe gastric distress.

Colon

The colon is a three to five-foot long thick, muscular organ, normally with an inverted u-shape. A typical person's colon is disfigured, with twists and kinks and prolapses which trap fecal material, leading to any and all colon problems, and autointoxication of the body's fluids. Many behavioral problems and epilepsy have been linked to colon toxemia and constipation. The colon is much more than a muscular tube; it has an intricate network of nerves which connect with every other organ and neuromuscular system in the body. (Refer to Figure 1 which shows a perfectly shaped colon.) The colon receives metabolic wastes from the small intestine. The colon also receives indigestible residue, including micronutrients, from the small intestine through the ileocecal valve. Muscular wavelike motion, peristalsis, moves the material forward as water and micronutrients are absorbed and stools are formed for elimination. A healthy colon has a slightly acid pH, and evacuation (bowel movements) normally occurs easily a short while after each meal.

In the absence of fiber or sufficient moisture in the residue, the peristaltic motion may be inefficient to move the material along, and constipation and mucoid matter buildup may result, leading to enervation and dysfunction of the colon. Fatigue and emotional upset also contribute to colon dysfunction. In times of irritation from a toxic overburden, the body may enact diarrhea, a massive elimination response. If there is not sufficient nerve energy to accomplish diarrhea, then wastes will accumulate, causing the condition of autointoxication, and this may lead to inflammation. Undigested food components passing into the colon, especially proteins from wheat, meat, dairy, legumes and nuts, are typically the major source of irritation because they decompose and their byproducts are toxic to the tissues.

The colon works symbiotically with bacteria (flora). There are two standard classifications of bacteria in the intestinal tract: healthful "friendly" bacteria (including lactobacillus bifidus and coli bacteria) and "unfriendly" coliform bacteria (including E. coli) which are actually misunderstood. As first demonstrated by biologist Antoine Béchamp in the mid-19th century, "unfriendly" bacteria are actually "friendly" bacteria which have mutated in the presence of toxic matter and serve the "friendly" function of eating (or cleaning up) the toxic matter.

"Unfriendly" bacteria are mistakenly blamed as the cause of illness. However, bacteria do NOT cause illness. Bacteria simply function to clean up wastes in the external and internal (bodily) environment. In the healthy colon of a person living on a 100% natural diet of fruits and vegetables, there may be a minimal amount of bacteria in the colon. In a SAD ("standard American diet") eater's colon, there may be as many as 400 species of bacteria, and sixty% of the wet weight of stools may be made up of bacteria. There are far more bacteria in a SAD eater's colon than the number of cells in our body. Some of the bacteria work symbiotically to maintain our health by manufacturing B vitamins and vitamin K, which is believed to help with blood clotting. Colons of SAD eaters have a huge population of putrefactive bacteria. We can create the condition of health and purity when we maintain a minimal population of only 100% healthful bacteria in the colon, and with that a perfectly healthy and strong colon.

Stools

"Stool" is a term describing the waste matter excreted from the bowel through the rectum, ranging in consistency from formed and hard (constipated) to watery (diarrhea). Stool characteristics are indicative of our diet, the effectiveness of our digestion and our level of health. Healthy people generally evacuate nontoxic stools, and bowel movements are barely noticeable and never unpleasant. Toxic stools are blatantly offensive to our senses, and their evacuation is typically difficult and tiring. Few people have ever eaten and lived healthfully (as taught herein and in other Natural Hygiene literature) and experienced healthy evacuation of nontoxic stools.

Toxic stools emit gases which are odiferously foul and offensive. Foul fecal gases or flatulence indicate that food has not digested completely; rather, it has decomposed (rotted or fermented) in the gut. The odors produced by decomposing nitrogenous proteins are characterized as "putrid." Odors produced by decomposing carbohydrates are characterized as "fermentive." The chemical byproducts (liquid and gaseous) of this rotting action include: ammonias, sulfides, histamine, tyramine, cadaverine, putrescine, indoles, skatoles and purines. Hydrogen sulfide, also referred to as "swamp gas," has the characteristic rotten egg odor which is common in sewer pipes. This gas is so corrosive that it eats through concrete piping, necessitating protective plastic liners. Imagine what it does to human flesh! All of these harsh chemicals irritate the bowel, leading to inflammation and, under chronic extreme conditions, the destruction and genetic alteration of cells, leading to polyps, tumors and cancer. They also circulate in the body causing systemic damage in a process called "autointoxication" which goes hand-in-hand with poor health. When the body's organs of elimination and self-purification mechanisms (known as the "immune system") are overwhelmed with toxins, we experience body odors and distress, leading to C&C in some people.

Diarrhea is an intelligent response enacted by the body when the contents of the bowels have reached a critically toxic level. The body sends water into the bowel and directs nerve energy to the bowel muscle to trigger peristaltic motion. Rapid evacuation of liquid feces is a sign of vigorous health-restorative detoxification. When the body enacts diarrhea, it is getting rid of threatening toxins. We want the body to get rid of the offending matter; we do not want to suppress diarrhea with medicines—that only adds to our toxic overload while further enervating our organism, extending the time it will take to heal.

When we have diarrhea, we must discontinue eating all fatty foods, rest, drink plenty of water and clear, fresh fruit juice, eat only health-supporting foods (if appropriate) and allow the body to complete its housecleaning job. Celery juice is the richest, safest and most natural source of electrolytes. Apple-celery and grape-celery juices are highly beneficial in this case. In cases of prolonged or extreme diarrhea with C&C, special care and guidance are required. This book presents general guidelines; however, each person needs a personalized healing plan to safely resolve his or her illness. In all cases of diarrhea, keeping oneself well-hydrated with water and juices is essential. If diarrhea is severe, your physician and a Hygienic Doctor, such as the author, should be consulted and blood testing should be performed to assess electrolyte levels.

Constipated stools are compact, low in water content and held together by mucous. If they float, they contain entrained gas. Constipation is a sign of incorrect eating and a lack of nerve energy needed for regular evacuation, that is, the bowel muscle is enervated to the point of inability to easily move digesta through the bowel. Many lifestyle factors can contribute to enervation of the bowel, as discussed later. In general, the top three factors are: 1. diets with foods too low in fiber and water content; 2. overeating cooked starchy and fatty foods; and 3. a deficiency of rest and sleep. Chronically compacted stools lead to irritation and, in some cases, disfigured colons (prolapses, hernias, strictures) and C&C because the fecal material stagnates, decomposes and its movement is difficult, fatiguing the bowel, rather than easily passing within 24 hours. The diet and healthful lifestyle program taught herein teaches the basic principles which enable the body to correct virtually all bowel problems and resume its normal shape and vitality.

As discussed in detail in the following sections of this book, there are several causes of food decomposition in the gut. They mainly fall under the categories of: 1. eating foods which are inherently indigestible; 2. eating foods in incompatible combinations; 3. eating too frequently; 4. eating when tired; 5. incomplete chewing.

When we eat incorrectly, exceeding the limitations of our digestive enzyme secretions and mechanical processing capabilities, food decomposes in the gut, as in a compost heap. That is, bacteria, yeast and, in some cases, parasites consume the nutrients and excrete wastes. This is nature's way of digesting or breaking down wastes, purifying our inner environment and recycling organic matter. The warm, moist, nutrient-rich environment of the bowel is an ideal fermenter of food residues. Weightwise, the bacteria content of the stools of people who eat mostly undigestible food matter is typically greater than the quantity of the solid residue itself. The higher the quantity of indigestible wastes in our bowels, the greater the population of bacteria and waste byproducts (gas, liquid and solid residues). The pH of toxic stool is typically acidic, indicating acid waste overload, as evidenced by rectal burning sensations. All these are undesirable and totally avoidable conditions. We need to eat in a way so that everything digests completely. We do not want to eat indiscriminately, creating the conditions for microorganisms to digest our food because that always results in poor health.

Ironically and sadly, most of what humans eat passes through the body undigested, poisoning their bodies and the environment. Human excrement is such an environmental pollution burden that humans have resorted to building sewage treatment plants. These costly plants serve to digest food residue which humans have not digested.

In wastewater engineering, the pollution strength of the sewage entering sewage treatment plants is measured as "biochemical oxygen demand" and expressed in units of "BOD." This quantifies the amount of oxygen required by aerobic microorganisms to decompose the degradable organic matter in a sample of sewage. The influent BOD is always very high. As such, the sewage is a pollution hazard and, if discharged untreated, would defile or even kill all life in a natural body of water. Within this scenario, bacteria and other microorganisma feast on the nutrients, multiply and pull oxygen out of the water, suffocating aquatic life while releasing metabolic wastes (swamp gas, etc.).

Sewage treatment plants employ aeration treatment processes wherein bacteria populations greatly multiply, consume the nutrients in the wastestream and reduce the solids volume. The remaining still-toxic sewage solids ("sludge") are separated out of the wastewater stream and typically sent to a landfill. The remaining wastewater is clarified, disinfected and discharged with a greatly-reduced BOD to the environment (creeks, rivers, oceans, meadows, agricultural fields, etc.). Septic tanks are sometimes used for individual home sewage treatment, employing an anaerobic rather than aerobic bacterial decomposition process, discharging BOD-reduced wastewater into the ground. In perspective, the home septic tank and the costly, inefficient and obnoxious sewage treatment systems are only necessary when humans eat foods for which they are not biologically suited. If we ate correctly, we would not need mechanical sewage treatment equipment to do the digestion job we were designed to completely accomplish in good health and with nontoxic results. Completely digested food from a healthy body in turn produces good "humanure" fertilizer for plant life. (Of course, "humanure" recycling is not entirely practical for city populations.)

When we eat correctly of only foods to which we are biologically adapted, as taught herein, the result is complete digestion, effortless evacuation, neutral or no stool or body odors, little or no flatulence and freedom from bowel disease. It is generally healthy to have one bowel movement per meal. For most healthy people, two or three bowel movements per day is normal. Bowel movements occur in seconds with no urgency and barely any sensation. Healthy stools are moist, formed and of fine, uniform consistency; they sink and crumble in toilet water with no signs of undigested pieces of food, mucous or blood; the pH is within the 6.7 to 7.3 range; their color resembles the food which was eaten in the previous meal, only slightly darker; there is no straining, long and difficult waiting, cramping, spasming, discomfort, offensive odor, stickiness, need for air deodorizers, shame or unpleasantness; there is minimal need for toilet paper and little or no gas. From a wholistic viewpoint, the end product of our digestion tells the story of how well we have eaten, digested our food and supported our health.

After you have detoxified, healed and mastered your dietary and lifestyle habits, the bowel will remain healthy and free of C&C and you will have the opportunity to enjoy optimal health and happiness in a clean and sweet-smelling body. You will feel well inside knowing that you've fully met the conditions required for everlasting health. That is our natural state of being and the happy, lasting outcome of healthful living.

Figure 1
Colon Illustration

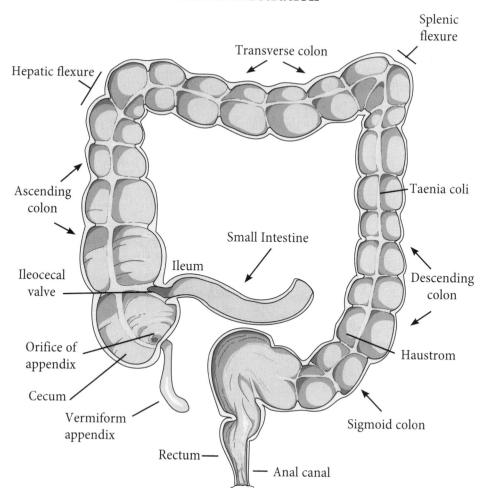

3.2
Bowel Hygiene

This section was extracted from *The Hygienic System. Vol. 1. Orthobionomics* by Dr. Herbert M. Shelton

Care of the Orifices of the Body

A truly healthy man is a clean being, internally. All of his excreta are inoffensive. The sweat from his body does not smell offensively. The discharge from his bowels has no offensive odor. His urine is not offensive. Offensive excreta are evidences of wrong food, wrong drink, lowered function and "disease." We do not get rid of such conditions by camouflaging them with perfumes, deodorants, etc. The discharge from the bowels should be odorless, aseptic (nonpoisonous) and should take on no odor upon standing.

Foul odors associated with the feces indicate lessened digestive powers, impaired secretion and decomposition of the food. The healthy digestive tract is clean and aseptic at all times. No fermentation occurs in it because normal secretions prevent this. But the more impaired the powers of life, the more fermentation takes place in the digestive tract and the worse is the odor of gases and solids excreted from the bowels. The same is true of the odors of the sweat, urine and breath. These latter, from the body of a sick man or woman, are at times almost unendurable. I have often wished for a gas mask while attending to a sick person because of the odors of the body and breath. The more decomposition that goes on in the intestines, the greater and more offensive will be the odors from the excreta of the body. The more meat and eggs, cheese, beans, peas, bread, potatoes, etc. one eats under such conditions of impaired function, the more offensive will be these odors.

If offensive odors come from your body, either from the mouth, kidneys, bowels, or skin, you are not enjoying the high degree of health that you are capable of enjoying. Your mode of living is not what it should be. You are filthy inside. If the odor is very bad, it indicates you are rotten inside.

Every organ in man's body acts automatically and in its own and the body's best interests. Every opening or cavity of the body which opens upon the outside world is self-cleansing.

Care of the Colon

It may be doubted whether any other organ in man's body is subjected to more abuse and is less understood than the colon. It is a constant object of solicitude and more effort is made to control the function of the colon than of any other organ.

Man's colon, like that of other primates, is designed as a reservoir for holding, for a few hours, the residue of fruits, roots, nuts and the indigestible seeds, skins, and fibers of vegetable foodstuffs—materials practically incapable of undergoing fermentation and putrefaction or giving rise to poisonous products of any kind.

When man became a meat and egg eater, he compelled his colon to deal with the putrescent residue of undigested eggs and flesh—highly offensive foods, which, when stored up in his colon for many hours, become a seething mass of putrefaction.

Urine stored in the bladder has already been eliminated. The kidneys have already removed this from the blood—it is out of the body and requires only to be voided. But in the case of the colon, we constantly mistake voiding for elimination. Matter that is in the colon, whether composed of food residues or waste matter excreted by the walls of the colon, is outside of the body—it requires only to be voided, not eliminated.

The walls of the colon excrete matter from the blood—they do not secrete matter into the blood. They form a "one-way street" and do not permit the much talked of absorption of poisons.

Bowel action is spontaneous and automatic. It does not require being forced or artificially regulated any more than does any other function of the body. We meddle with bowel function too much. "But doctor, aren't you going to do anything to make my bowels move?" asked a young lady of me once. I replied: "Your bowels do not require being made to move any more than your heart needs to be made to beat or your lungs to breathe. The trouble with your bowels now is that they have been made to move too much, already."

This lady, whose age was twenty, had taken laxatives and cathartics every day of her life from infancy. We let her wait upon nature. On the thirteenth day her bowels moved, and in a few days they were moving twice a day on two meals a day. This has continued for several years.

Bowels act when there is necessity for action. There are many ways of forcing increased action of debilitated organs for a brief period, providing there is enough power in reserve to produce the action, but these things always and necessarily diminish the power of that action and do so precisely to the degree to which they accelerate the action. The increase of action is occasioned by the extra expenditure of power called out, not supplied.

The normal bowel movement, which only empties the rectum, should not consume more than five to ten seconds. No effort should be required; no straining and grunting are necessary. The movement is free and easy and so quickly over that one hardly realizes he has had a movement. It is accompanied by a distinctly pleasurable sensation. The stools should be free of all odor; they should be well-formed and neither soft nor hard.

Small ribbon-like stools indicate spasticity of the rectal sphincters. Large hard stools mean delay in emptying, with distention of the rectum. Foul stools represent decomposition. Watery stools mean diarrhea or other abnormality. The color of *the stool, though usually yellow, will be determined by the food eaten. Spinach and beets, for instance, both give the stools characteristic colors.*

The colon is an integral part of the body. Its function is efficient or not, depending upon the support it receives from the general system. If health is impaired, bowel function will be impaired. If health is good, bowel function will be good. We should place the emphasis upon general health—upon wholeness and integrity.

Few people realize how much time and money they really spend trying to cover up evidences of their ill health instead of improving their health. If they are constipated, they blame the constipation for their ill health instead of blaming the impairment of their health for the constipation. This leads them to try to improve their health by using cathartics and laxatives to force their bowels to act, instead of overcoming their constipation by improving their health. Constipation is an effect, a symptom—not a cause. It is good health that insures daily bowel movements and not daily movements that insure good health. The best rule for dealing with the bowels is to attend to your own business and let the bowels attend to theirs.

3.3
WHOLISTIC FACTORS
IN COLITIS AND CROHN'S DISEASE

Although C&C have specific local symptoms, health care is best when performed in a wholistic context. When a health disorder is manifesting, the causative factors must be identified and then eliminated. There are many factors which determine our health and contribute to C&C. It is necessary to identify and address all of them in each case. They fall under the broad headings of mental, emotional, environmental, musculo-skeletal and dietary. We can observe and learn from animals in nature which do not get C&C. We should live as closely to the laws of nature as possible, simplify our lives and diets, and eat only clean digesting vegan (non-animal) foods to enable our bodies to heal.

What follows is a brief overview of some of the main contributing factors of C&C. Dietary factors, the major focus of this book, will be addressed in greater depth in the following section.

Genetics

Our inherited genes may play a role in susceptibility to C&C, but our genes certainly do not cause C&C. If a person with C&C has parents or other relatives who have had C&C, this does not mean that C&C cannot be permanently overcome. Our diets, emotions, environment and lifestyle factors are the most significant factors in C&C.

Lack of Sleep

A lack of quality sleep leads to chronic fatigue and the breakdown of our health. The majority of healing takes place when we are asleep. Extra sleep is what everyone with C&C needs. Ten hours minimum is recommended. More than ten hours is better. When we sleep, the body is able to replenish its stores of nerve energy. It is nerve energy which powers self-healing. When we are awake and active, our nerve energy is being depleted. When we close our eyes, nerve energy recharges the body with energy for self-healing. As such, quality sleep and closed-eye rest are essential elements of self-healing.

Thoughts and Beliefs

Certainly, every one of us has been ingrained with erroneous beliefs about the cause and nature of disease, about how to care for ourselves, what and how to eat, and whom to turn to for help when we become ill. These beliefs were handed down from our family, teachers and society and it is crucial to identify the errors of our ways and live healthfully.

It has been said that we are what we think. Indeed, our thoughts and beliefs shape our reality, including our health. They can drain our energy and stagnate our bowels, impairing elimination and setting up C&C. Our mind and body are one; therefore, what we think affects our body in profound ways. In order to heal and establish health, thoughts and beliefs which do not serve us must be identified and no longer held. This is a process of self-awareness whereby we step into a new health-minded persona. We need to cease thinking unhealthful thoughts and cease sending any unhealthful messages to our body, especially our gut. Thoughts of shame, blame, hate, anger, resentment, hopelessness, fear, etc. which produce "bad," painful or depressed feelings need to be identified and we need to disengage from them. A skillful counselor who is grounded in a somatic awareness approach, such as The Diamond Approach, can help with this process. (See www.ridhwan.org.)

To train our mind, it is useful in the beginning to feed ourselves healthful thoughts, especially ones concerning our gut, and to consciously release thoughts which are not constructive. Incorrect beliefs need to be identified and released as well. Via the teachings in this book and other books on Natural Hygiene, as well as counseling sessions with a Hygienic health education professional, the reader can learn to let go of erroneous beliefs and become instilled with accurate beliefs about health. The more we practice healthful thinking, the easier it becomes and the healthier we become.

Emotions and Lack of Vitality in the Belly

Many if not all people with C&C have deep-rooted, unresolved emotional issues which contribute to their illness. This is common in modern society, even in people who appear to be healthy. Emotions are energy patterns of the body—they are expressive gifts of life. Having emotional issues is nothing to be ashamed of. In fact, our emotions help protect us and deepen our life experience.

Our gut is our "personal power center" and the colon is a very emotionally alive organ—it is connected with our feelings. Some people channel feelings of anger, sadness and/or fear into their gut and subconsciously hold on, contracting the flow of vital nerve energy to the bowel, leading to incomplete elimination and toxicosis. Some have deep-rooted, shameful feelings about their bowels. If we harbor unhealthy feelings about our bowel functions, then we will not be sending healthy messages to our gut. Each of our organs and cells needs to receive positive energy and healthy, loving messages from our minds in order for us to create and maintain good health. We need to breathe fully, accept and release our emotions and maintain relaxed emotional poise in order to promote complete digestion, elimination and bowel health. With improved diet and digestion and clean elimination, new happy feelings and better health will emerge.

Facing our emotional issues is often difficult; we need to be gentle on our-selves when addressing our emotional health needs. The sure path to colon health is to work on accepting and then embracing all of our emotions, while learning to disengage or "witness" our emotional persona. As we accept our emotions, we are more readily able to release them and live in the flow of life. When we are ready to work on our emotions, it is highly recommended to work with a counselor or therapist skilled in guiding clients through emotional resolution.

One's emotional healing path is a lifelong journey involving many "teachers." When seeking a professional helper, it is important to find someone with whom you deeply resonate. The relationship between the client and counselor is crucial. When a trusting bond is developed, old emotional wounds can be resolved, re-patterned, or healed most effectively. Emotional resolution (or healing) ultimately leads to better health, as self-love grows and one gives his or her body the kind of care it needs and deserves.

Social Stressors

Social pressures, e.g., pressure to work extra hard to get ahead at any cost, have lead many college students and professionals to "burn themselves out." Sometimes the individual's weak link is the bowel, and C&C manifests. Those who have difficulty managing stress, or those who internalize stress, tend to get C&C. When we are stressed, the environment in our colon can change dramatically— the colon tends to contract and become enervated, and friendly bacteria die as the colon's pH becomes highly acidic. Eating heavy comfort foods when we are stressed is hazardous, because when we are stressed the digestive system shuts down and food does not digest properly, decomposing into toxic matter which irritates the colon, leading to digestive disorders and C&C.

Meditation, yoga, tai chi, other exercise, music, visualization tapes, nature outings, extra sleep, nutritious diet, health support groups, stress counseling and belief and thought re-patterning are examples of tools that can help with stress.

Environmental Stressors

These stressors include air, water and electromagnetic pollution and residues on food from pesticides, processing and preserving chemicals. As many as 400 different pesticides are approved for use in the commercial growing of food crops, and tens of thousands of chemicals are used by food processors in the prepara-tion of their food products. Many if not all of these substances can cause cellular damage and neuro-hormonal disturbances leading to nervous disorders, bowel disorders and cancer.

Breathing smoggy, oxygen-deficient city air can contribute to irritability and impaired digestion. Drinking chlorinated city water can deplete the population of "friendly" bacteria in the colon.

Pet hair or dander, mold/fungus and seasonal pollen blooms are potential allergens to be avoided. Vapors from chemical household cleaners, perfumes and cooking can also irritate the system.

Maternal Smoking

A study has shown that both passive smoke and maternal smoking at birth are significantly associated with the development of C&C in children.

Drugs and Laxatives

Antibiotics, anti-inflammatories such as cortisone and prednisone, and azulfadine (sulfa) drugs destroy intestinal flora. Anti-inflammatories may also cause lesions in the intestinal lining and increased permeability under prolonged use. Sulfa drugs destroy many vitamins and some contain an aspirin component which is destructive to tissue. Using these drugs to suppress general inflammation may serve to temporarily hide local symptoms, but they have the effect of further deteriorating a person's health. Antacid abuse may also be a contributing factor in C&C. Alcohol and caffeine are extremely toxic substances which deplete nerve energy as they leach valuable minerals out of our bodies, and their habitual use can contribute to C&C—they must be discontinued in order for healing to take place and health to be maintained. Laxatives work by irritating the bowel. Their use can cause over-stimulation of the muscles, enervation, sluggish bowel tone and further constipation.

Yeast, Parasites, and Increased Intestinal Permeability

An overgrowth of the intestinal yeast candida albicans ("candida") is an increasingly common condition which can have a ravaging effect on the bowel. Yeast overgrowth begins in a colon which has an abnormal pH, and the yeast byproducts exacerbate a toxic condition (toxicosis). The yeast actually takes root in the intestinal wall and scavenges the tissue. Studies have shown that yeast overgrowth can cause increased intestinal permeability (or "leaky gut") which correlates with the incidence of C&C. With increased permeability, the protective mucousal barrier is breached, allowing the absorption of potentially injurious macromolecules into the bloodstream. This creates a greater burden on the organs of purification and elimination, systemically contributing to fatigue, allergies and C&C. In addition to yeast, parasites, putrefaction, fermentation, free radicals and anti-inflammatory drugs can also contribute to increased intestinal permeability and C&C. A whole foods vegan diet with juicy fruits and plenty of fresh vegetables will help reestablish an acidic bowel pH and reverse yeast conditions.

Lack of Exercise and Incorrect Posture

Exercise helps stimulate peristalsis, provides oxygen which is needed for good digestion, and is essential in maintaining strong muscle tone in our abdominal organs. Exercise is also essential for relieving stress and enhancing emotional balance. Lack of exercise can lead to sluggish bowel function which can contribute to C&C. The body cannot rebuild itself without physical stimulation including aerobic exercise. People who are ill and fatigued need rest (not exercise) in order for the body to replenish its vital energies. Once healing has begun and bodily energies are on the rise, a gentle exercise program is recommended. Exercising to the point of fatigue must be avoided.

Lower back stiffness and incorrect spinal alignment can greatly reduce the flow of nerve energy to the abdominal organs. Yoga, stretching and other forms of physical therapy such as chiropractic care may be essential for overcoming C&C.

Shallow or Incorrect Breathing

With free and deep breathing, the diaphragm will massage and tone up the abdominal organs and emotions are more readily released. With shallow breathing, the organs can lose their tone and ability to function properly. When breathing correctly, the abdomen expands and air is delivered deep into the lungs for efficient distribution to the abdominal organs. When breathing incorrectly, the reverse happens—the abdomen is expanded upon exhaling and carbon dioxide remains in the lower part of the lungs and may diffuse to the abdominal organs, causing oxygen starvation and enervation. It is always beneficial to practice deep rhythmic breathing upon awaking and after each meal.

Ileocecal Valve Malfunction

The ileocecal valve functions to allow the passage of digested material from the small intestine into the colon. The valve opens when food enters the stomach. If the valve is bound up with constipated material or enervated from autointoxication, the valve may remain open. This can allow the passage of incompletely digested material into the colon, causing bacterial decomposition to produce excessive gas, leading to irritation and then C&C. Some chiropractors and massage therapists can manually close an open valve, but dietary changes and stretching or yoga may help it resume its normal function.

Enemas and Colonics

When an individual has C&C, enemas and colonics are not recommended because the colon needs a rest (not an invasive, unnatural cleansing), and the water pressure can force toxins into the system causing toxic shock. When we are in any health condition, enemas and colonics are risky and not recommended—they wash out bacteria which work symbiotically with the bowel to keep it healthy. The unnatural eliminative reflex action is enervating to the colon muscle and nerve system, which can lead to a sluggish, constipated and disfigured bowel. Colonics stir up toxins which can enter the bloodstream, resulting in acute illness and distress. It is best to allow the colon to detoxify naturally. Contrary to popular belief, as confirmed by any gastroenterologist, fecal matter does not accumulate and adhere to the colon walls as plaque which can only be eliminated via therapeutic means (such as colonics, enemas and colon cleansers). The high-water content diet recommended herein will enable the body to evacuate stagnant digesta and feces from the entire bowel safely and naturally in short time.

Other Enervating Practices

The following habits also deplete nerve energy, lowering vitality and possibly contributing to C&C: excessive exercise; swimming in chlorinated water; excessive sex; saunas; acupuncture; lack of vacation and relaxation time.

4
VEGAN DIET PLAN

4.1
DIETARY FACTORS IN COLITIS AND CROHN'S DISEASE

There are a few (but not enough) books, studies and case histories with personal testimonials about people who have naturally overcome C&C by making dietary changes and discontinuing the use of medicines. In addition, the author of this book has helped over 1,000 such people heal. In each case, the individual switched from the SAD, which is heavy in meat and refined flour products, to a vegan whole foods diet high in water content. People who have switched to natural, vegan whole foods diets have found that their previous diet was largely responsible for their C&C and that medicines only contributed to their ill health. They also discover that their new natural diet is more satisfying and energizing because it is "the real thing"—it is pure, nourishing food which their taste buds truly appreciate the most. The following is a discussion of key dietary factors in C&C.

Deficient Nutrient and Fiber Intake

The Standard American Diet (SAD) is largely deficient in basic nutrients and trace minerals, and this may be a major factor in the development of digestive disorders. We need to eat a diet rich in essential and trace minerals in order to carry out digestive functions. Digestive enzymes are made by the body from the nutrients we eat. A person who has C&C is probably losing the building blocks of enzymes at a fast rate, causing digestion to worsen.

Raw food, that is uncooked fruits and vegetables, is our natural food, and when we introduce it to our nostrils and palate, our senses immediately recognize it and secrete the proper digestive enzymes. Raw food furnishes us with friendly bacteria and fiber necessary to maintain healthful bacteria in the colon. When properly masticated, raw food is most nourishing. Fiber is also available from cooked whole foods such as vegetables; however, cooking breaks down the fiber and destroys bacteria. Friendly bacteria and fiber play major roles in keeping our gut healthy. Fiber provides bulk which allows the peristaltic wave to move digesta toward elimination. Without sufficient fiber, the intestinal muscles have to overwork and can become enervated. Fiber also absorbs the toxins which may contribute to C&C.

Insufficient Chewing

Chewing may have the greatest impact on digestion of any single factor. The digestive process begins in the mouth with the secretion of digestive enzymes and moistening and mastication of food. The chewing motion of the jaw sends signals to the hormonal system, triggering the flow of digestive juices and digestive nerve energy. The masticating action of our teeth breaks open plant fibers, releasing nutrients. Ptyalin, an enzyme necessary for digesting starches, is secreted only in the mouth. Chew your food slowly and thoroughly, mixing the food with your salivary enzyme secretions. Solid food must be chewed until thoroughly liquefied. Hurried eating, or eating when tired, tend to result in the swallowing of chunks of unchewed food, creating digestive problems. With thorough chewing—30 to 60 chews per mouthful—the burden on the digestive organs is greatly reduced, indigestion will diminish, and nutrient uptake and bowel health will improve.

Excessive Cooked Food in the Diet

by Dr. T. C. Fry

In nature all animals eat living foods as yielded up by nature. Only humans cook their foods and only humans suffer widespread sicknesses and ailments. Those humans who eat mostly living foods are more alert, think more clearly, sharply and logically and become more active. Best of all, live food eaters become virtually sickness-free!

Cooking is a process of food destruction from the moment heat is applied to the foodstuff. Long before dry ashes result, food values are totally destroyed. If you put your hand just for a moment into boiling water or on a hot stove, that should forever persuade you just how destructive heat is. Food is usually subjected to these destructive temperatures for perhaps half an hour or more. What was living substance becomes totally dead very rapidly with exposure to heat!

Cooking renders food toxic! The toxicity of the deranged debris of cooking is confirmed by the doubling and tripling of white blood cells after eating a cooked food meal. The white blood cells are the first line of defense and are, collectively, popularly called "the immune system."

As confirmed by hundreds of researches cited in the prestigious National Academy of Science's National Research Council's book, Diet, Nutrition and Cancer, *all cooking quickly generates mutagens and carcinogens in foods.*

Proteins begin coagulating and deaminating at temperatures commonly applied in cooking, and are devoid of nutritive value.

Vitamins are rather quickly destroyed by cooking.

Minerals quickly lose their organic context and are returned to their native state as they occur in soil, sea water and rocks, metals and so on. In such a state they are unusable and the body often shunts them aside where they may combine with saturated fats and cholesterol in the circulatory system, thus clogging it up with cement-like plaque.

Heated fats are especially damaging because they are altered to form acroleins, free radicals and other mutagens and carcinogens as confirmed in Diet, Nutrition and Cancer.

Thus you can see that dead foods make dull, diseased and sooner dead people.

Poor Food Combining

Food combining is a practice which everyone can benefit from. It helps the body completely digest foods so that no more internal poisoning occurs. The author recommends that everyone follow food combining guidelines.

Foods may be categorized according to the specific types of digestive enzymes and transit times they require in the digestive system. Refer to the food combining chart in Figure 2. In basic terms, there are six food categories: fruits, proteins, fats/oils, carbohydrates, non-starchy vegetables and mildly starchy vegetables.

An example of a good food combination is fruit eaten alone or with neutral greens (such as lettuce) and/or celery and/or cucumber. Fruit needs to digest and absorb quickly and will not do so if eaten with starches or proteins—gastric distress will ensue under unfavorable digestive conditions. When eaten properly on an empty, clean stomach, ripe fruit is the easiest food of all to digest—it is already predigested in the ripe form.

Another good combination is proteins (e.g., nuts which require acidic digestive juices) with non-starchy vegetables (e.g., lettuce, celery or cucumbers which require neutral digestive juices).

Yet another good combination is starches (e.g., corn, squash, potatoes, whole grains) with non-starchy vegetables (e.g., lettuce, celery or cucumber which require neutral digestive juices). Starches require the secretion of alkaline digestive juices/enzymes (e.g., ptyalin and amylase) and proteins require acidic digestive juices/enzymes (e.g., hydrochloric acid, pepsin and trypsin). When we have starchy and proteinaceous foods and the corresponding alkaline and acidic digestive juices mixing together in the stomach, the result is poor digestion and toxemia—the alkaline and acidic digestive enzymes cancel each other out, rendering them ineffective as the starches ferment and the proteins putrefy. This is why meat and bread and potato eaters have putrid bowels, and why they tend to develop C&C and cancer. For a person who has seen his or her health deteriorate with C&C, proper food combining is invaluable for improving digestion.

Overeating and Bingeing

A chronically overloaded and overworked bowel is a stressed bowel. This will enervate the bowel, leading to toxemia, irritation then inflammation. Stagnant bulk will decompose in the bowel, poisoning the tissues and, eventually, lead to distress. Excessive roughage from such items as grains, raw vegetables , raw nuts and raw seeds can irritate a healthy bowel and scrape and exacerbate an inflamed bowel, worsening C&C.

If food is eaten on a too frequent basis, then previous digestion may be suspended and incomplete, causing it to decompose and toxify the bowel and bloodstream. If the body is required to focus its energies on digestion all day, the bowel (and entire body) can become chronically fatigued, further impairing digestion. Many foods require several hours to travel through the system for proper digestion. Furthermore, time is needed between meals to allow for assimilation and metabolic balancing.

Bingeing, an eating disorder stemming from emotional issues, can also have an enervating effect leading to C&C. Most people associate food with comfort. This association is natural since our earliest memories connect food with warmth and nurturing. In addition, some foods, e.g., creamy or fatty foods, relax or sedate us, shifting our mood and thoughts. Many people seek to dull or cover up painful emotions by filling up with food, and this pattern is not easily broken. As such, those who start to make dietary and lifestyle changes with the best of intentions may find themselves sliding back to old patterns of eating more than they sense their bodies can handle. Some people even binge until they are too full to eat another bite, preferring this uncomfortable physical condition which covers up their usual painful emotions. These habits often create more stress, both physical and emotional, when the person harshly berates himself for the behavior. Such compulsive eating does not warrant self-punishment.

For someone who eats compulsively, trying to rigidly limit one's diet to certain items at first often leads to backlash and rebellion. It may be best to take a gradual transitional approach, changing the diet as one is ready. Generous amounts of compassion, support, patience and nurturing are needed. Working with a skilled and trusted somatically-oriented therapist, team, or group which provides deep emotional support and healing is highly recommended. People who suffer from C&C are sensitive, gifted people. As these qualities are encouraged in a safe environment, the person can come into balance and compulsive behaviors will cease to rule dietary habits.

Irritants, Allergens and Stimulants

Onions, leeks, radishes, mustard, garlic, chile peppers, vinegar, salt, salty condiments and most spices are irritating to the bowel and contribute to and exacerbate C&C—they must be discontinued. Certain drugs, such as aspirin, irritate the stomach and bowel. Molds and certain chemical food additives are allergenic, and they are all toxic and can contribute to C&C. Grain gluten, an undigestable protein commonly found in wheat, is another irritant which can cause C&C.

Caffeinated drinks, especially coffee, all spices, salts, many herbs and drugs, high-protein supplements, "super food" supplements, "energy drinks and bars," all other exotic dietary supplements, most manufactured food products, alcohol, tobacco and marijuana are toxic stimulants which deplete our energy, unbalance our system and rob our health. All must be avoided.

Salt

Avoid all salt—it's a toxic, irritating, corrosive, stimulating, enervating and potentially deadly poison. Yes, even Celtic and Himalayan salts are destructive to your body and health—don't be fooled by marketing hype! These inorganic substances may be trendy but they are not healthful. In addition to sodium chloride, they contain numerous toxic elements including heavy metals, such as aluminum, cadmium, lead and mercury. These wreak havoc in the body, and are very difficult to eliminate.

If you live in a northern region or near the ocean, you have probably seen how rock salt and salt spray eat steel members and chrome coatings on automobiles. If you've ever had an open flesh wound and exposed it to salt, your senses will have told you how destructive it is. Salt paralyzes the intestinal villi and kills cells— would you knowingly bathe your delicate villi, your arteries, veins and capillaries with such a corrosive solution? Salt brine kills insects and "pickles" vegetables. Do you want to run a solution of that through your brain 24 hours a day? An ounce of salt, taken all at once, spells suicide.

You cannot become healthy if your sense of taste is befuddled by unnatural flavorings. Salt does not bring out the flavor of food; it overpowers your taste buds, deadening them to all sensation other than additional salt, causing unnatural cravings, overeating and beverage guzzling.

Salt bonds with water, and its toxicity necessitates extra fluid intake. The body's dilution response causes the cells to become dehydrated, severely impairing health. Salt also throws off the blood's electrolyte balance (for example, the sodium to potassium ratio), eroding health and impeding healing. Most illnesses cannot be overcome when salt is part of the diet. The salt eaters I've counseled did not heal their C&C until they followed my recommendation of giving up salt.

Hypertension (high blood pressure), edema, cardiovascular disease, stroke, atherosclerosis, asthma, arthritis, rheumatism, Alzheimer's disease, lupus, premenstrual syndrome, gout, cancer and a host of other disease conditions are linked to salt. Can the body handle a little bit of salt? Maybe, but not on a regular basis. It's not worth the risk.

We do need mineral salts, no doubt about it. Where should we get our mineral salts? Plant foods is the natural answer. The liquids from fruits and vegetables contain all of the mineral salts we need, in safe, organic, usable form. For rich, satisfying flavors, obtain produce grown in soil generously mineralized with a rock powder amendment. If possible, grow your own produce, adding such mineral sources as rock powder, azamite or kelp powder to your compost and soil.

Abstain from salt, clean out, eat whole, fresh, ripe, raw, organic tender vegetables plus savory and sweet fruits. In one to two weeks your salt cravings will vanish and unseasoned foods will taste outrageously delicious.

Mucous Formers/Constipators

Foods may be categorized as mucous-forming and non-mucous-forming. In general, cooked foods, especially meat, dairy, beans including soy and grains are mucous-forming; fresh fruits and vegetables are non-mucous-forming. Mucous formers have been shown to be the source of constipation and play a major role in many disorders including C&C. The body secretes mucous to protect its sensitive tissues from unnatural harmful substances. In a healthy person who eats a natural diet of fruits and vegetables, there is no or very little mucous, and it is light and clear. The body of a person who consumes meat, dairy and flour products will have thick and often foul-smelling mucous secretions, accumulations and body fluids, and with that, constipated feces.

Constipated feces are packed together with mucous and do not easily pass out with normal elimination. Constipation develops in the colon as water is drawn out of matter containing mucous. Some colon health books report that the average person has as much as 10 pounds of this hardened matter in his or her bowel. Without a change to a non-mucous-forming diet, this matter will continue to accumulate and can contribute to C&C and cancer.

Acid-forming Foods

The human body must maintain its fluids at a slightly alkaline pH in order to survive. Neutral pH is 7.0; acid pH is below 7.0; alkaline pH is above 7.0. The bloodstream pH must be maintained within a pH range of 7.35 to 7.45; blood pH outside that range results in death.

The term "pH" means "potential hydrogen." Substances in aqueous solution are determined to be either alkaline or acidic according to their predominance of hydroxyl (OH-) versus hydrogen (H+) ions. Hydroxyl ions are negative and alkalizing; hydrogen ions are positive and acidifying. The pH scale is logarithmic. This means that each pH point below 7.0 is ten times times more acidic than the next higher value. For example, pH 5.0 is ten times more acidic than pH 6.0 and 100 times more acidic than pH 7.0. Likewise, pH 9.0 is ten times more alkaline than pH 8.0 and 100 times more alkaline than pH 7.0.

Acidifying factors include: 1. acid-forming foods; 2. exercise; and 3. stress (mental and emotional).

Metabolic waste acids are produced in every cell. This requires a sufficient reserve of alkaline minerals in the body for their neutralization. Under normal conditions, acid wastes are minimal and easily neutralized and transported to the organs of elimination. Our kidneys are adept at eliminating excess alkaline minerals.

When faced with excessive acidifying factors, the body must work extra hard to buffer the acid wastes, preserve alkaline homeostasis and eliminate acid wastes from the bloodstream, cells, tissues and organs. Extreme, chronic acid waste loads force the body to resort to buffering the acidity with its limited reserve of calcium, its most abundant alkalizing mineral reserve, which is mostly stored in the bones. This undesirable condition is the leading cause of osteoporosis. Attempting to thwart osteoporosis with calcium-rich foods which contain predominantly acid-forming minerals, such as milk, cheese and fish, actually causes further osteoporosis. A chronic acidic condition ("acidosis") constantly stresses the body, resulting in weak electrochemical energy conduction, low bio-energetic vibration, physical and mental enervation, debilitating disease (including C&C), physical degeneration, rapid aging and death.

The primary acidifying (or acid-forming) dietary factors are as follows:
- any and all animal foods and products: meat (including fish and fowl) and dairy (butter, cheese, cream, eggs, milk and yogurt),
- all grains and flour products except amaranth, millet and quinoa,
- all beans/legumes except fresh lima beans, fresh peas, green beans, soybeans and sprouted beans/legumes,
- all nuts and seeds except almonds, chestnuts, fresh coconuts, pine nuts (pignolias) and sesame,
- white sugar, high-fructose corn syrup, and some other sweeteners,
- carbonated soft drinks,
- coffee,
- alcoholic beverages,
- processed sugar.

Drugs, marijuana and tobacco are also acidifying.

Except for blueberries, cranberries, plums and prunes, all raw fruits and vegetables are alkaline-forming (or alkalizing). Alkalizing foods promote high biochemical conduction and sustained vibrant health. Extreme alkalinity, or "alkalosis," is a rare condition. Except for serious health failure, such as end-stage cancer, only in the instance of kidney failure could alkalosis be an issue, and even then there would be other far more serious issues to contend with. The alkalosis at that point would be a symptom, not a disease. Thus, it is apparent that a diet of predominantly fruits and vegetables is safe, health-promoting and should comprise the bulk of our diet.

Foods are not classified as acidifying or alkalizing based on the pH of their juices in the raw state. For example, oranges, limes, pineapples, peaches and tomatoes contain acidic juices; however, they are not acid-forming but, rather, they are alkalizing on the basis of their alkalizing mineral composition and metabolic end reaction. Their acidic juices are easily diluted and neutralized by our alkaline digestive secretions before they enter the bloodstream.

Foods are determined to be acidifying/acid-forming or alkalizing/alkaline-forming on the basis of their metabolic end reaction in our body. That means after the nutrients from a food are utilized in the cells the resulting waste fluid pH is either acidic or alkaline. This is a function of each food's mineral composition. Certain minerals create acidity in aqueous solution; others create alkalinity. Foods with predominantly acid-forming minerals impart acidity to the cells and metabolic waste stream. Foods with predominantly alkaline-forming minerals impart alkalinity to the cells and metabolic waste stream.

The primary acid-forming minerals are: phosphorus, sulfur, chlorine, iodine, bromine, fluorine, copper and silicon. The primary alkaline-forming minerals are: calcium, magnesium, sodium, potassium, iron and manganese.

The following information was extracted by permission from the book *Composition And Facts About Foods And Their Relationship To The Human Body* by Ford Heritage, published by Health Research:

Alkalinity-Acidity of Foods in Metabolic Reaction

After foods are eaten they are oxidized in the body, resulting in the formation of a residue or ash. In this residue, if the minerals sodium, potassium, calcium and magnesium predominate over sulfur, phosphorus, chlorine and un-combusted organic acid radicals, they are designated as "alkaline ash" foods. The converse of this is true for foods designated as "acid ash."

Numerical values of alkalinity or acidity were determined in long, painstaking analytical laboratory work. The concentrations of the various elements were determined separately and then computed in terms of equivalents. The excess at one group of minerals over the other is expressed as cubic centimeters of normal acid or base (alkaline) per 100 grams of edible food. The values obtained are called degrees of acidity or alkalinity.

Most Alkaline Reaction
43.7 *Fig, dried*
41.6 *Lima bean, dried*
36.6 *Apricot, dried*
25.3 *Raisin*
20.4 *Swiss chard*
20.3 *Prune, dried*
17.5 *Dandelion greens*
16.4 *Soybean sprouts*
15.8 *Spinach*
15.0 *Taro corms and tubers*
14.2 *Cucumber*

14.0 *Lima bean, fresh*
13.5 *Almond*
12.1 *Peach, dried*
11.1 *Beet*
10.7 *Avocado*
10.5 *Kale*
10.4 *Chive*
10.2 *Carrot*
10.2 *Rhubarb*
9.9 *Endive (escarole)*
9.6 *Date*
9.1 *Chestnut*

8.6 Parsnip
8.5 Granadilla
8.5 Lemon with peel
8.5 Coconut meat, dry
8.5 Rutabaga
8.4 Onion, mature dry
8.3 Tomato, ripe
8.2 Peach, fresh
8.2 Plum
8.1 Celery
8.1 Watercress
7.7 Blackberry
7.7 Guava
7.7 Lemon
7.7 Bamboo shoots
7.7 Iceberg lettuce
7.5 Cantaloupe
7.5 Coconut milk
7.4 Loganberry
7.4 Pea, dried
7.3 Sweet cherry
7.3 Leek
7.2 Potato
7.1 Orange
7.0 Lettuce: Cos, Loose-leaf
6.7 Prickly pear
6.7 Sweet potato
6.6 Apricot, fresh
6.5 Turnip
6.4 Grapefruit
6.2 Nectarine
6.2 Common cabbage
6.0 Banana
6.0 Coconut meat, fresh
6.0 Kohlrabi
5.8 Pineapple
5.7 Raspberry
5.7 Tangerine
5.5 Gooseberry
5.0 Mango
4.9 Quince

4.9 Mushroom
4.8 Sapodilla
4.8 Snap bean
4.8 Radish
4.5 Orange juice
4.5 Eggplant
4.5 Okra
4.3 Brussels sprout
4.2 Broccoli
4.2 Horseradish, raw
4.1 Sour red cherry
4.0 Lemon juice
3.9 Red cabbage
3.5 Pomegranate
3.4 Pear, fresh
3.2 Cauliflower
3.2 Chicory
3.2 Pumpkin
2.8 Winter squash
2.7 Grape
2.7 Savoy cabbage
2.6 Strawberry
2.2 Apple
2.2 Watermelon
1.8 Sweet corn
1.3 Pea, fresh green
0.1 Olive oil
Least Alkaline Reaction

Neutral Reaction

Least Acid Reaction
0.1 Asparagus
0.2 Chinese water chestnut
0.8 Sorghum grain
1.4 Blueberry
2.1 Filbert
2.3 Cress
3.2 Brazil nut
3.8 Olive, green pickled
4.3 Artichoke, globe

4.3 White bean, dried
7.8 White rice
8.5 English walnut
10.3 Jerusalem artichoke
10.5 Lentil
10.6 Peanut

10.9 Wheat grain
11.3 Rye grain
Most Acid Reaction

Grains

Grains are not digested well by humans. In their natural form they are hard and unpalatable. Their major caloronutrient component is comprised of starch which is complex carbohydate—clusters of many molecules, requiring a relatively great amount of chemical action to break their bonds for use as caloric fuel. Starch must first be enzymatically digested by our salivary digestive juices into simpler sugars, then further reduced by additional enzyme secretions from the pancreas (in the duodenum). Because this process takes hours and humans are not designed to secrete copious quantities of the starch-splitting enzymes, starches typically ferment in the gut, generating alcohol and vinegar, causing excessive mucous production, irritation and toxemia.

Fermentation is the bacteriological decomposition of carbohydrates. Natural fruit sugars and starches can ferment in the stomach and small intestine under certain conditions of improper eating, insufficient secretion of digestive enzymes, and/or reaction with accumulations of internal debris. The byproducts of fermentation are lactic acid, acetic acid (vinegar) and alcohol. Similar to the byproducts of putrefaction, these toxins can lead to autointoxication, as evidenced by sour stomach, body odors, gas, fatigue, "food drunkenness" (or attention deficit disorder—"ADD") and then C&C.

Starches are low in water and, thus, tend to cause constipated, mucousy stools. Except for amaranth, millet and quinoa, grains are acid-forming. Many grains contain gluten, an undigestible, irritating protein which is a prime culprit in C&C. Excess starch consumption causes hyperglycemia (elevated blood sugar), causing the body to store the excess carbohydrate as fat, leading to obesity while overworking the pancreas and causing diabetes.

Refined grain products, especially those made from flour, along with some whole grains, all sugary syrups, dried fruits and white potatoes cause the highest rise in blood sugar level. "Glycemic Index" is a ranking system for carbohydrates based on their effect on blood glucose levels. Grain products (bread, pasta, rice, cereal, baked flour products) rank in the high glycemic index category, while some whole grains and most whole fruits rank in the medium glycemic index range. However, as author David Mensosa explains on his web page www.mendosa.com/gilists.htm, glycemic index is an inadequate tool for assessing the blood sugar load imposed by various carbohydrate food sources. He shows that the "glycemic load" of foods is a better indicator of blood sugar elevation. While the glycemic index only indicates how quickly sugar enters the bloodstream, glycemic load accounts for the rise with respect to the quantity of carbohydrate per each food item. Because grains, grain products, potatoes, syrups and dried fruit are low in water and high in carbohydrate content, those foods impose a much higher glycemic load than do fruits, which average 85% water and much lower carbohydrate content by weight. Calculating glycemic load based on the quantity of carbohydrate per 100 grams of food, grains and grain products rank two to four times higher in glycemic loading than do juicy fruits.

High glycemic load foods cause metabolic chaos leading to diabetes, fat storage, candidiasis (candida albicans fungal condition), constipation, attention deficit disorder, fatigue and a host of other problems. As such, whole fruits, which are far more easily digested and smoothly metabolized than grains, are our most healthful source of caloric sustenance.

In his book *Grain Damage*, Dr. Douglas Graham cites these and a dozen other reasons not to include grains in our diet. Our conclusions are that grains hinder healing and ripe, sweet, whole fruits are the premium food, carbohydrate fuel source and health-promoting food for humans, especially those with C&C.

Are we designed to eat grains? That is, are we graminovores? Dr. T. C. Fry answered the question thusly:

Graminovores are creatures that subsist on grains and/or cereals. Being graminovorous means we live from grasses and grass seeds, though grass eaters are really called herbivores. Strict grain eaters are called graminovores. Many birds in nature live on grass and weed seeds. Grass seeds include wheat, oats, rye, barley and rice which were developed by human mastery of nature only within the last 10,000 years. There are thousands of other grass seeds that occur throughout nature.

Of course, we'd all reject grass seeds as items of diet in nature. First, they are in a condition we can neither masticate nor digest, being heavy on starches. We would gag on the equivalent of a spoonful or two. You might try a mouthful of wheat berries without husks removed as you must eat them in nature—that won't work for us. Further, if you ate a tablespoon of raw flour made from grass seeds (cereal grains), you'd gag.

As grass seeds neither attract, tantalize nor arouse us in their raw natural state, we can reject them as natural human fare even though most of the human race presently consumes grains. Thus, we are not natural graminovores.

Are we starch eaters? To test this question I will not ask you to do the impossible, i.e., take a hand full of grass seeds (presuming you could gather them in nature) and start chewing. Or, try a spoonful of flour of any grain. You'd choke up on the first spoon of it as your starch license (salivary amylase) would be speedily exhausted. This would amply prove to you that we were not starch eaters in nature when we had not mastered fire. Instead of being a palate-tingling delight, starches are a tortuous affair.

When humans can freely eat starchy roots, grains and tubers such as cassava, taro, potatoes and wheat in their raw state to satiation and proclaim the experience a gourmet treat, then both you and I might concede that we're starch eaters.

In *The Health Reporter, Volume 1, Report No. 3* published by Life Science, my associate Marti Fry wrote the following article:

Starches Are Second-rate Foods

Have you noticed how often we state that fruits are the foods to which we are biologically suited? We rank them as first-class foods and we rank starchy foods such as tubers, legumes and grains as second or third-class foods. One reason for this, as you may know, is that most starchy foods have to be cooked to make them tasty. Of course there are exceptions to this:

1. Some people like potatoes, yams, etc., raw.

2. Some mildly starchy vegetables, such as carrots, peas and cauliflower, are palatable in the raw state to most people.

3. Many legumes can be sprouted instead of cooked.

But despite these exceptions, starchy foods are not ideal for humans. Unlike sugars from fruits, which pass almost directly from the stomach to the small intestine for absorption, starches must be converted to sugar for the body to unlock their energy potential.

Most animals secrete starch-splitting enzymes called "amylases," derived from the Latin word meaning "starch-splitting." In humans, starch digestion begins in the mouth: our saliva contains an amylase called "ptyalin," derived from the Greek word "ptyalon" meaning "saliva." Ptyalin, also called salivary amylase, chemically changes starch into maltose, a complex sugar. Many other animals, such as pigs, birds and other starch eaters, but not humans, secrete other additional amylases to insure complete starch digestion. To be sure of adequately digesting the starch we humans consume, we must chew our food very, very thoroughly so it becomes well-mixed with saliva.

The starch that's converted to maltose by salivary enzymic action is further broken down in the small intestine by the enzyme maltase into the simple sugar, dextrose, for the bloodstream can absorb only simple sugars, never starches nor complex sugars. (Dextrose is dextrorotatory glucose.)

Only 30 to 40% of the starch eaten can be broken down by ptyalin in the mouth. If starches are eaten with (or close in time to ingestion of) acid fruits (citrus fruits or tomatoes) or with protein foods, the ptyalin in the saliva that's swallowed with the food cannot further break down the starch into simple sugars.

This is because ptyalin can only act in an alkaline environment, and the stom-

ach environment becomes acid when proteins are consumed. The acids in fruits will also inhibit the secretion of ptyalin. Hence, you should take care to eat starchy foods (if you eat them at all) with vegetables and not with acidic or high-protein foods to insure the best possible digestion. We do secrete a pancreatic amylase in our intestine to digest starches not handled by salivary amylase (ptyalin). But starches often partially decompose in the stomach before they get to the intestine.

In addition to the often disagreeable taste of raw starchy foods, there's a problem relative to human starch digestion which leads people to cook or sprout them. According to The Textbook of Medical Physiology by Arthur C. Guyton, M.D.:

"Most starches in their natural state, unfortunately, are present in the food in small globules, each of which has a thin protective cellulose covering. Therefore, most naturally-occurring starches are digested only poorly by ptyalin unless the food is cooked to destroy the protective membrane."

If cooking can destroy the protective membrane around the starch cells, what is it doing to the food's value? Cooking changes the minerals and proteins into unusable forms and destroys most vitamins!

Chewing only partially breaks the protective covering of starch globules and so raw starches can only be partially digested. While undigested foods cause pathogenic problems in the human body, the toxins ingested when we eat cooked foods (with deranged vitamins and minerals) cause even greater problems.

In light of how the human body uses starches by changing them to simple sugars through a complicated and only partially effective process, why not consider getting all your carbohydrate needs from fresh fruits which are already in the form of simple easily-digestible sugars? We don't need starches at all and can thrive more healthfully without them.

Overeating of Fats

Excessive fat consumption is the number one causative factor in almost every major Western disease condition. Cooked fatty foods, including mainly animal meats and derivatives, dairy foods (milk, eggs, cheese, butter) and oils (which are essentially liquid fat) are most destructive to human health and a prime cause of C&C. As Dr. Douglas Graham states in his thoroughly researched book, The 80/10/10 Diet, when humans consume more than ten% of their calories in the form of fat—in the cooked or raw state—health deteriorates. Most Americans and other peoples consuming a meat-based diet derive a huge 40 to 60% of their total caloric intake from fat.

Furthermore, as documented in the landmark yet widely ignored book Diet, Nutrition and Cancer, heated fats are carcinogenic. As such, every bite of a cooked fatty food, or the refined oil component, is a deadly affair. The higher the cooking temperature, the more carcinogenic the result. Fried oils are the worst offenders with regard to cancer as well as C&C. The typical result of fried oil consumption is severe diarrhea accompanied by internal inflammation, triggering or exacerbating C&C.

Fats and oils are highly perishable. As such, they may be rancid before eaten or may rancidify in the system if not properly digested and eliminated. This results in the formation of free radicals which have a ravaging effect on mucous membrane cells, possibly contributing to C&C.

People with C&C must discontinue the intake of all fatty foods—cooked and raw—during the healing phase in order to restore health.

In response to the question "Are we fat eaters?", Dr. T. C. Fry wrote:

In nature there are very few fats we can get in any quantity without violating our biological disposition. Avocados, durians, olives, coconuts, nuts and seeds are heavy on fats. Avocados and durians furnish fats in a predigested state when ripe. Coconuts furnish fats as monoglycerides/glycerols before they set their fats as triglycerides in a storage form. Coconuts are, therefore, in the jelly-like state, easily digested. When matured and hardened, it is almost impossible to digest them.

Broccoli and cauliflower have considerable fatty acids in an easily usable state when eaten in the raw, fresh condition. However, they have some unwanted toxic sulfur compounds. We get predigested fats adequate to meet our fatty acid needs from fruits. An occasional avocado or seeds and nuts are quite satisfying.

Those who subsist substantially on fats do not do well. Eskimos are very short-lived. They consume about 200 grams, about 1,800 calories, daily. Their short-lived condition is probably more attributable to their heavy protein consumption than fats. They consume about 200 grams of protein daily incidental to their fat-eating and this places a great burden upon their organs, especially liver and kidneys. Because of the acid-forming properties of metabolized proteins, Eskimos lose their teeth at an early age and suffer severe osteoporosis. Eskimos are eaters of animal fats and proteins, primarily as derived from fish. Be it noted that, during the berry-picking season, Eskimos are said to eat only berries during the short season they are ripening.

Biologically, we are not a species of fat eaters, but incidental eaters of fats. Fruits that have lots of fat are predigested so that we handle them with ease when they are ripe. Other forms of fat require hours for their digestion, quite atypical of fruits to which we are most favorably disposed. Fats may lie in the small intestine several hours before bile is secreted into it with which to emulsify them, thus exposing them to lipases which reduce them to monoglycerides (fatty acids) and glycerols.

I adjudge that we are not a species of fat eaters except incidental to our fruitarian disposition.

Protein Putrefaction

The major food protein sources are animal products, beans, legumes, seeds, and nuts. All of these are typical sources of putrefaction, especially when eaten in meal-size quantities. Putrefaction, actually a fermentation process, is the bacteriological decomposition, or rotting, of nitrogenous foods or proteins in our gut which occurs under certain conditions of incorrect eating and insufficient secretion of digestive enzymes. Putrefaction of proteins proceeds easily at body temperatures, just as milk will spoil on a warm day. In our society, the putrefaction of meat and dairy products (except yogurt, which is partially digested by bacterial cultures in its preparation) is the major culprit in that regard. The byproducts of putrefaction include ammonias, sulfides, histamine, tyramine, cadaverine, putrescine, indoles, skatoles, and purines—all toxic compounds which poison the body and mind, leading to rapid aging, fatigue and disease. The body has a limited capacity to eliminate these. If some of these toxins should get into the blood, it is the liver's job to neutralize them. However, when elimination is not complete, such as in cases of constipation or when the liver is impaired, these toxins will cause autointoxication and are typically a major factor in C&C.

Addressing the question "Are we protein eaters?", Dr. T. C. Fry wrote:

To hear the exponents of the meat trust, you'd think we're in imminent danger of disease and death if we fail to eat meat three times a day. The truth is that eating meat three times daily will cause the very conditions we're taught to fear. We're in no danger of protein deficiency unless we're eating a 100% cooked food diet. On the other hand, there are grave dangers in eating cooked proteins. At normal cooking temperatures, proteins are coagulated, deaminated and largely oxidized. The nitrogenous materials are soil for putrefactive bacteria. The carbohydrate portions of cooked proteins are usable for caloric values but still present the problems that cooked carbohydrates pose.

If we must eat proteins, we must eat them raw to derive their full benefit. But proteins, per se, are not created as food. They are created by plant and animal life as components of organisms, seeds, enzymes, ova, etc. Most proteins of this nature have toxic protective compounds. The bean family has anti-enzyme factors. Eggs have avidin. Nuts also have anti-enzyme factors. Seeds of peaches, apples and many other fruits have hydrocyanide. Humans do not secrete the enzymes to negate or break down these toxic substances.

From fruits we derive as much protein as is present in mother's milk for a growing baby! Moreover, fruit proteins come to us predigested as do other ripened fruit components. There are many alarmists who warn us about protein deficiencies of fruits and many other presumed deficiencies. If we developed in nature on fruits to our high state as anthropologists have found, then the real deficiencies are in the thinking of those who proclaim deficiencies. Their evidence is usually based on researches with pathological specimens, especially those whose metabolic and assimilative faculties are very impaired. They base their thinking from a standpoint of disease rather than health, from a modality and curing mentality rather than a correction of pathogenic practices. In saying that our natural foods are deficient, they are simultaneously proclaiming improvidence in nature. Or, in effect, saying: "God, you made a terrible mistake in providing for us and especially in giving us a sweet tooth." Advocating the consumption of proteins and yet more proteins when those so advising know by their own researches and knowledge that the proteins will be cooked and contribute to heavy pathology is nothing less than criminal.

One more consideration: If we ate only proteins in their raw state we'd quickly become diseased and perhaps even suffer death! Why? Because various amino acids require from about 60% to 137% of their carbohydrate energy potential for their deamination and utilization. The net result would be starvation. That's one reason so much weight is lost by the obese on protein diets. And the intoxication that results from putrefaction is the reason so many of these dieters become diseased, with some dying.

Are we protein eaters? Emphatically, no!

Animal Meats

Meat (any animal flesh, including fish) is the single most causative dietary factor with C&C. The author has never seen or heard of a case of complete and lasting healing of C&C where the person continued to eat meat. Dead animal foods do not bring life to sick people. They cannot because meat is mostly indigestible and it poisons the bowel, bloodstream and tissues while acidifying the body and undermining our health. Even infrequent meat eating can trigger a flare-up of C&C. Meat and dairy products of any kind are not essential to the human diet, and their use has been directly correlated with the major diseases prevalent in Western society, including C&C and colon cancer. All of the nutrients which are essential to maintaining peak health and longevity are available from plant sources. Animal products are acid-forming, mucous-forming, high in fat, devoid of fiber and low in water content; they require great amounts of energy to digest, and usually putrefy in the bowel, creating an overload of "unfriendly" bacteria and toxic byproducts. When the body is too acidic from acid-forming foods, it will not be able to heal C&C until detoxification has occurred. When fats are cooked using high heat, free radicals are created which are known to cause cancer. Many people with C&C are lactose-intolerant, meaning they cannot digest milk sugars. In every case this author has seen, people do not overcome C&C until they stop eating meat and dairy products. Eating a diet high in cooked animal products destroys most people's health, and it is advisable to eliminate all animal products from their diet: beef, pork, fowl, fish and dairy. When we stop eating animal products, we immediately liberate a great amount of physical energy which the body can use for detoxifying and healing itself.

In response to the question "Are we carnivores?", Dr. T. C Fry wrote:

A carnivore is an eater of carnage or flesh. This does not accurately portray animals said to be carnivores. Animals that live on other animals usually consume most of the animal, not merely the flesh. True carnivores lap the flowing and oozing blood of their prey with relish. They delight in the guts and its partially digested contents. And they will consume the bones and gristle (collagen or cartilage). Dogs, for instance, require about 1,700% as much calcium as humans, for animal flesh is extremely acid-forming. Blood and bones are required to offset the acidotic end materials. They also require about 1,200% more protein than humans. When you note the relish and gusto with which dogs go for whole animals, you can be sure that what carnivores need for their nourishment is quite delicious to them.

Do you relish the idea of crushing the life of a rabbit with your bare hands and teeth? Can you lick its blood with gusto, getting it over your face, hands and body? Would you dig into its guts with pleasure? Would you love to chew on its bones and gristle? Would you love to swallow chunks of its flesh, not being fastidious about swallowing hair and vermin that might be involved? Would you like to do the same for any plant-eating animal that you could apprehend, kill and consume while still in its warm and fresh state?

Of course, you and every unperverted person loves animals as fellow creatures on earth. Killing them is repulsive to you and eating them in the freshly killed state is even more disgusting to you. Yet, most of us do consume flesh and some organ meats while rejecting blood, bone, most fats and the entrails or offal. But we kill our animals by proxy. We denature and derange flesh and organs with heat and camouflage it with condiments. Does this describe a carnivore to you? Would you, in a state of nature, relish chasing down animals and eating them? Again, this is alien to your natural disposition and actually sickening.

True carnivores also secrete an enzyme called uricase to metabolize the some 5% uric acid in flesh. We secrete none and thusly must neutralize it with our alkaline minerals, primarily calcium. The resulting calcium urate crystals are one of the many pathogens of meat-eating, in this case giving rise to or contributing to gout, arthritis, rheumatism and bursitis.

Are humans natural meat-eaters? There are too many considerations in physiology, structure (miscalled anatomy), aesthetic disposition and psychology that characterize us as non-flesh eaters to even seriously entertain such notions.

I had a nutritionist tell me in front of an audience that we had canine teeth and that proved our meat-eating character. I responded with: "You really mean dog teeth, don't you? Like fangs?" This caused her to redden. Then I related one of Abraham Lincoln's favorite retorts: "If you counted a sheep's tail as a leg, how many legs would it have?" Invariably the answer was "five". To which Lincoln would respond: "Only four. Counting the tail as a leg doesn't make it one."

I think you'll agree that we are not equipped in any aspect of our being as carnivores.

Addressing the question "Are we milk drinkers, that is, are we sucklings of animals?", Dr. T. C. Fry wrote:

I doubt that humans ever directly suckled cattle, goats, mares, camels, sheep and other animals. And, of course, the idea of doing this is obnoxious to our disposition. I refer, facetiously, to milk eaters as secondhand grass eaters although, to be sure, grass has all the nutrients necessary to support life.

While we can live on milks (certain Africans like the Masai live substantially on milk and blood, thus reducing themselves to parasite status), these are by no means our natural foods. Milk-drinking as a regular part of our intake is only a few hundred years old, with the exception of certain Arabic and African peoples.

Milk-drinking is pathogenic. If milk and milk products were discontinued today, millions of people would cease to suffer sicknesses and pathologies within a short period. In fact, if this alone was discontinued, the hospitals would virtually empty out and physicians' waiting rooms would be mostly vacated.

Milk-drinking is also an act by proxy. If we had to get milk directly from the teats of animals by suction, I'm sure we'd skirt milk altogether. I would and I'm sure you would, too.

The following is an excerpt from the extensively researched book *The Undigestible Truth About Meat* by my colleague Dr. Gina Shaw, M.A., A.I.Y.S.:

Did you know that the two leading causes of death in the U.S. are directly related to the consumption of meat? When I use the term "meat," in order to clear up any confusion anyone may have, I am referring to all animal flesh, be it from cows, turkeys, pigs, chickens, fish, in fact, any animal that lives and breathes and that humans consume! I am talking about all animal flesh.

Patrice Green, J.D., M.D. and Allison Lee Solin state that animal products easily account for our largest intake of pesticides and herbicides, in fact, more than 80 to 90% by some estimates.

Meat also has antibiotic residues. One half of all antibiotics in the U.S. alone are used in the production of livestock. Antibiotics, too, can contribute to hormone-disruptor exposure.

As if that isn't enough, in a recent article entitled "Meat Your Death?" by Lawrence J. Jacobs, M.D. and Caroline Kweller, they report that a survey by Public Citizen, the Government Accountability Project, and the American Federation of Government Employees, found that 46% of federal inspectors had been unable to recall meat laden with animal feces, vomit, metal shards, and other contamination.

In 1998 USDA (United States Department of Agriculture) declared safe for human consumption animal carcasses carrying a host of diseases, such as cancers, tumors, open sores, poultry pneumonia, infection arthritis, and diseases caused by intestinal worms.

Food borne diseases such as campylobacter, listeria, E. coli, and salmonella affect millions of Americans and Britons each year and kill more than 5,000, particularly children, the elderly, and those with weak immune systems. In the vast majority of cases, people contract these diseases after eating animal products-meat, poultry, eggs, and dairy or from items contaminated by animal products or animal feces.

Animal food is highly acid-forming and, according to Dr. Robert Young, a microbiologist and nutritionist from the U.S., has high levels of bacteria, yeast/fungus and associated toxins.

Cooked animal foods are dead, enzymatically speaking. They lack enzymes which help us to break down foodstuff, they lack phytonutrients which are by their very nature abundant in fresh, raw plant foods and they lack many essential vitamins and minerals.

In a recent report by Dr. Green and Ms. Solin, they argue that organic meat, dairy and eggs certainly cannot be held to be a healthy option as not only do animal products contain cholesterol, and are typically high in fat, they have been found to significantly raise risks for heart disease, stroke, hypertension, obesity and cancer.

Meat is the most putrefactive of all foods. This means that meat is more liable to decay in the human gastrointestinal tract than any other food. Flesh, when it is eaten by humans, tends to undergo a process of decay in the stomach or intestinal tract causing a poisoning of the blood. Putrefaction in meat-eaters is evidenced by bad breath, heartburn, eructations and smelly stools, and it is probable that the attempts of the body to eliminate these wastes has a profound influence on the shortening of our life span.

If the body fluid that bathes our cells is overloaded with waste, an excessive secretion of bile, fatigue, weakening and aging are the inevitable results. The accumulation of toxic substances in the body causes the deterioration of the intestinal flora and the blood vessels gradually lose their natural elasticity—their walls become hardened and thickened. Irreversible damage to the organism will then inevitably occur.

The hardest thing for the human body to digest is cooked animal protein—it leaves us feeling very weak and tired. Protein, being the most complex of all food elements, makes its utilization the most complicated. Those people with impaired digestion will find it preferable to ingest a lesser quantity of concentrated protein which they will be more capable of utilizing, rather than a greater quantity which not only cannot be processed efficiently, but which may poison the body.

When protein is eaten in greater amounts than the body is capable of utilizing, the organism is subjected to the toxic byproducts of protein metabolism, which it has been unable to eliminate—and the inevitable result is degenerative disease.

Meat passes very slowly through the human digestive system, which is not designed to digest it. In fact, flesh foods can take about five days to pass out of the body (plant foods take about one day). During this time the disease-causing products of decaying meat are in constant contact with the digestive organs. The habit of eating animal flesh in its characteristic state of decomposition creates a poisonous state in the colon and wears out the intestinal tract prematurely.

Often, poisonous bacteria present in flesh foods are not destroyed by cooking, especially if the meat is undercooked, barbecued, or roasted on a spit—these are notorious sources of infection. The stomach will attempt to break down animal flesh with chemicals which are ill-equipped to handle flesh foods as we have such a low amount of hydrochloric acid, as compared with carnivorous animals. This hydrochloric acid we do have is also low in acidity, as compared to a carnivorous animal. Next, the animal flesh passes into the small intestine until it comes to the ileocecal valve. Passing through the ileocecal valve, it enters the cecum which is at the base of the ascending colon. From here the second stage of digestion starts. The chyme becomes a seething mass of intestinal flora. When dead bodies are incorporated in our food, the flora is putrefactive and their mission is to destroy. From the colon, they are drawn into the bloodstream by suction and, as they circulate around the body, disease or sickness is the inevitable result. On a fruit and vegetation diet, the natural flora are fermentative and break down this type of food—they are not pathogenic and are quite harmless to the body for the simple reason that we are not flesh eaters.

British and American Scientists who have studied intestinal bacteria of meat-eaters as compared to vegetarians have found significant differences. The bacteria in the meat eaters' intestines react with digestive juices to produce chemicals which have been found to cause bowel cancer. This may explain why cancer of the bowel is very prevalent in meat-eating areas like North America and Western Europe, while it is extremely rare in vegetarian countries such as India. In the US, bowel cancer is the second most common form of cancer (second only to lung cancer). Conversely, recent studies have found that chicken meat is the most carcinogenic meat that people can eat due to the amount of the carcinogen PhIP contained in it—although, as we will find, all meat is dangerous and carcinogenic to the human body.

Another important point is that meat contains waste products that the animal did not get to eliminate, and toxic hormones and fluids released into the bloodstream and tissues at the moment of the death of the terrified animal. The cells continue to produce waste materials which are trapped in the blood and decaying tissues. The nitrogenous extracts which are trapped in the animal's muscles are partially responsible for the flavor of the cooked meat. Just before and during the agony of being slaughtered, the biochemistry of the terrified animal undergoes profound changes. During times of intense rage or fear, animals, no less than humans, undergo profound biochemical changes in dangerous situations. The hormone level in the animal's blood—especially the hormone adrenaline—changes radically as they see other animals dying around them and they struggle futilely for life and *freedom. These large amounts of hormones remain in the meat and later poison the human tissue. According to the Nutrition Institute of America, "the flesh of an animal carcass is loaded with toxic blood and other waste byproducts."*

Therefore, toxic byproducts are forced throughout the body, thus poisoning the entire carcass. The flesh is invaded by a putrefactive virus which are nature's scavengers which function to get rid of dead bodies. As soon as an animal is killed, proteins in its body coagulate, and self-destruct enzymes are released (unlike slow decaying plants which have a rigid cell wall). Soon denatured substances called ptomaines are formed. Due to these ptomaines that are released immediately after death, animal flesh and eggs have a common property—extremely rapid decomposition and putrefaction. By the time the animal is slaughtered, placed in cold storage, "aged," transported to the butcher's shop or supermarket and purchased, brought home, stored, prepared and eaten, one can imagine what stage of decay one's dinner is in. According to the Encyclopedia Britannica, *body poisons, including uric acid and other toxic wastes, are present in the blood and tissue.*

Cholesterol is mainly found in animal products. Meat, fish, poultry, dairy products and eggs, etc., all contain cholesterol, while plant products, on the whole, do not. Choosing lean cuts of meat is not enough; the cholesterol is mainly in the lean portion. Many people are surprised to learn that chicken contains as much cholesterol as beef. Every four-ounce serving of beef or chicken contains 100 milligrams of cholesterol. Most shellfish are very high in cholesterol. There is no "good cholesterol" in any food.

Colon cancer is acknowledged to be the predominant type of cancer in the United States, and it is the second leading cause of cancer mortality. An article in the Wall Street Journal several years ago tells about a study of colon cancer by Dr. William Haenzel, Dr. John W. Berg and others at the National Cancer Institute. Dr. Berg said: "There is now substantial evidence that beef is a key factor in determining bowel cancer incidence."

Scientists have reported evidence that two characteristics of meat-based diets are specific influences in colon cancer:

1. Fecal transit time: a low-fiber diet allows carcinogens to be concentrated and held in contact with the bowel mucosa for long periods, while a high residue diet (a vegetarian diet) produces more rapid passage of body waste.

2. Influence of the diet on the amount of carcinogens produced by the body: it has been found that meat fat tends toward production of carcinogens in the intestine.

Let us now examine the charge that flesh-eating is supposed to be a superior source of protein. Well, upon examining the evidence, the truth is exactly opposite! The effects of encumbering our bodies with the proteins of other animals serve to promote diseased conditions of the human organism. Dr. Herbert M. Shelton wrote that allergy and anaphylaxis (a kind of toxic shock of the tissues) are not mysterious and that they are due to long-standing poisoning of the body by excess or inappropriate protein foods. Animal proteins are often not reduced to their constituent amino acids, but are absorbed in more complex form. Absorption by the body of such partially digested proteins poisons the human body and so-called "allergic symptoms" may result in gout, arthritis, cancer, or any one or more of a host of degenerative diseases.

One of the favorite arguments of flesh-eaters is that proteins from the plant kingdom are "incomplete," because, they say, no plant food contains all of the twenty-three identical amino acids. Studies of man's physiology and the effect of his consumption of foods from plant kingdom have shown conclusively that it is not necessary to consume all of the amino acids at one sitting, or even the eight (some references say ten) essential amino acids that are not fabricated within the body. Foods we eat are processed by the body, and the amino acids, vitamins and minerals, and other nutrients reserved in a pool for later use as needed. When we eat, we replenish the reserves in this pool, which is then drawn upon by cells as and when required. We do not live upon one protein food, but upon the protein content of our varied diet, which provides all of the protein needs of the body. Guyton's Guidance Textbook of Medical Physiology *is authority to this important information. The book shows that amino acids are picked up from the bloodstream and cells of the body.*

Dr. Hoobler, researching at Yale University, demonstrated the superiority of nut protein. It was he who proved conclusively that the protein of nuts not only provides greater nutritive efficiency than that of meat, milk and eggs, but that it is also more effective than a combination of these three animal proteins. Fruits and vegetables, although containing relatively smaller amounts of protein in their natural state, are excellent sources of supplementary amino acids for complete and optimal nutrition. The protein in raw nuts and seeds, and in uncooked fruits and vegetables, are readily available to the body, and are therefore said to be of high biological value. During the process of digestion, the long chains of amino acids (the building blocks of protein) are gradually broken up for the body's use in synthesizing its own protein (as any species must do). However, when proteins have been cooked or preserved, they are coagulated. Enzyme resistant linkages are formed which resist cleavage, and the amino acids may not be released for body use. In this case, the protein is useless and/or poisonous to the body, becoming soil for bacteria and a poisonous decomposition byproduct.

Since the nutrients available from raw food are several hundred% greater than those available from food that has been cooked or otherwise processed, and since flesh foods are usually not eaten raw and whole by humans, this in itself would be an important reason why firsthand protein foods from the plant kingdom, which may be eaten uncooked, are superior .

Nowadays, many people eat fish rather than beef in the hope of limiting fat and cholesterol; however, many fish including catfish, swordfish, and sea trout contain almost one-third fat (saturated fat also contributes to degenerative disease). In fact, salmon is fifty-two% fat and, ounce for ounce, shrimps have double the cholesterol of beef. The Physicians Committee for Responsible Medicine argue that fish and fish oil capsules contain an unhealthy amount of artery-clogging saturated fat and that studies show that diets based on fish do nothing to reverse arterial blockages. Moreover, blockages continue to worsen for patients who regularly eat fish. Fortunately, eating vegetables such as broccoli, lettuce and beans provides essential fatty acids in a more stable form, with zero cholesterol and little saturated fat—a much healthier substitute!

Contrary to the myths that chicken and turkey (and fish) contain less cholesterol and that, reportedly, chicken and turkey represent a good option for those on a healthier diet, Dean Ornish, M.D., reported that on a five-year follow-up of patients on his popular plan for reversing heart disease with a totally vegetarian diet, compared with patients on the chicken and fish diet recommended by the American Heart Association (AHA), the majority following the AHA guidelines got progressively worse, whilst those who made intensive changes got progressively better.

Kieswer stated that too much protein also puts a strain on the kidneys, forcing them to expel extra nitrogen in the urine, increasing the risk for kidney disease. Also, the combination of fat, protein and carcinogens found in cooked chicken creates troubling risks for colon cancer. Chicken not only gives you a load of fat you don't want, its heterocyclic amines (HCAs) are potent carcinogens produced from creatine, amino acids and sugars in poultry and other meats during cooking. These same chemicals are found in tobacco smoke and are fifteen times more concentrated in grilled chicken than beef. HCAs may be one of the reasons that meat-eaters have much higher colon cancer rates: about three hundred% higher compared to vegetarians.

Dr. Neal Barnard of the Physicians Committee for Responsible Medicine, in reviewing recent research findings, stated that it has long been known that cooked red meat contains cancer-causing heterocyclic amines, which form as the meat is heated, but the U.S. National Cancer Institute has shown that oven-broiled, pan-fried or grilled/barbecued chicken carries an even bigger load of these carcinogens than does red meat. In fact, they argue that chicken is far more cancer-causing than red meat (the number of PhIPs in a well-done steak contains about 30ng/g, but grilled chicken reached 480ng/g). These dangerous chemicals are strongly linked to colon cancer, but may also contribute to breast cancer. Conversely, Dr. Barnard also mentions that the cholesterol content of chicken is actually the same as that of beef, and the fat content is not much different, either.

As previously mentioned, vegetarians have lower rates of colon cancer than non-vegetarians (Phillips, 1980). Incidence of colon cancer has been strongly linked to the consumption of meat (Armstrong, 1975). Willett (1990) carried out a study of over 88,000 women aged between 34 and 59 years. The study found that women *eating red meat daily ran over twice the risk of developing colon cancer than women eating red meat less than once a month. Reduced incidence of colon cancer in vegetarians may be attributed to dietary differences which include increased fiber intake, increased consumption of fruit and vegetables, and decreased intake of total fat and saturated fat.*

The mechanism by which a vegetarian diet is protective against colon cancer is unclear and a great deal of research is being carried out in this area. It has been suggested that secondary bile acids are carcinogens, which may play an important role in colon cancer. These are derived by bacterial metabolism from primary bile acids made in the liver and secreted into the intestine. Vegetarians have lower levels of secondary bile acids than non-vegetarians (Turjiman, 1984). The differences in bacterial populations between the intestines of vegetarians and non-vegetarians may also be important. Bacterial flora in vegetarians has been shown to possess reduced ability to transform bile acids into potential carcinogens.

The role of dietary fiber in prevention of colon cancer may also be important, as was first noted in 1971 when it was suggested that the high incidence of colon cancer in Western countries was linked to low fiber diets. Other dietary components associated with high fiber foods have also been implicated as having protective effects.

Leukemia is the overproduction of white blood cells to contend with toxic materials in the blood, due to the byproducts of protein breakdown. As you are probably aware, leukemia is a type of blood cancer and, as such, the causes (a meat-based diet) would inevitably be the same as for the causes of cancer (above). Dr. Paul Kouchakoff discovered, in his extensive experiments, that cooked meat causes a tremendous proliferation of white blood cells in the bloodstream—the increase is two to four times that of normal proliferation! The body produces white blood cells in order to surround toxic particles and to escort them to the nearest exit point, usually the kidneys.

Leukemia is always associated with an extremely high amount of uric acid in the blood. Uric acid is an inevitable byproduct of meat consumption, as mentioned in the first chapter. In fact, animal products are comprised of approximately 15% uric acid!.

Diverticular disease affects the colon. It occurs frequently in Western countries, where intake of dietary fiber is low. Gear (1979) found diverticular disease to be less frequent in vegetarians, twelve% of vegetarians had diverticular disease, compared with thirty-three% of non-vegetarians. This is thought to be due to the increased fiber of vegetarian diets.

The China Project on Nutrition, Health and Environment was a massive study involving researchers from China, Cornell University in Boston, and the University of Oxford researching the relationships between diet, lifestyles and disease-related mortality in 6,500 Chinese subjects from 65 mostly rural or semi-rural counties. The rural Chinese diet is largely vegetarian or vegan, and involves less total protein, less animal protein, less total fat and animal fat, and more carbohydrate and fiber than the average Western diet. Blood cholesterol levels are significantly lower. Heart disease, cancer, obesity, diabetes and osteoporosis are all uncommon. Areas in which they are becoming more frequent are areas where the population has moved towards a more Western diet, with increasing consumption of animal products. The China Health Project has clearly demonstrated the health benefits of a diet based on plant foods. One of the project's coordinators, Dr. T. Colin Campbell of Cornell University, stated: "We're basically a vegetarian species and should be eating a wide variety of plant foods and minimizing our intake of animal foods."

Research shows that adding fire to food causes dangerous changes in the food structure, including the creation of carcinogenic substances. According to research performed by cancerologist Dr. Bruce Ames, professor of Biochemistry and Molecular Biology at The University of California, Berkeley, various groups of chemicals from cooked food cause tumors: nitrosamines are created from fish, poultry or meat cooked in gas ovens and barbecues, as nitrogen oxides within gas flames interact with fat residues; hetrocyclic amines form from heating proteins and amino acids; polycyclic hydrocarbons are created by charring meat; mucoid plaque, a thick tar-like substance, builds up in the intestines on a diet of cooked foods. Mucoid plaque is caused by uneliminated, partially-digested, putrefying cooked fatty and starchy foods eaten in association with high-protein flesh foods; lipofuscin is another toxin: an accumulation of waste materials throughout the body and within cells of the skin, manifesting as age-spots, in the liver as liver spots and in the nervous system, including the brain, possibly contributing to ossification of gray matter and senility.

From the book Diet, Nutrition and Cancer published by the Nutritional Research Council of the American Academy of Sciences (1982) and the FDA (Food and Drug Administration) Office of Toxicological Sciences, carcinogens in heated foods include: hydroperoxide, alkoxy, endoperoxides and epoxides in heated meat, eggs, fish and pasteurized milk; ally aldehyde (acrolein), butyric acid, nitropyrene, nitrobenzene and nitrosamines from heated fats and oils; indole, skatole, nitropyrene, ptomatropine, ptomaines, leukomaines, ammonia, hydrogen sulfide, cadaverine, muscarine, putrecine, nervine and mercaptins in cheese.

Raw food is the optimum diet for humankind. Fired foods lose their nutrient content by up to 80% and their protein usability by approximately 50%. Cooking also destroys 60 to 70% of the vitamins, up to 96% of vitamin B_{12} and 100% of many of the lesser factors, such as gibberellins, anthrocyans, nobelitin, and tangeretin, which boost the immune system and other body functions. According to Dr. Paul Kouchakoff, every time we eat cooked food, our bodies produce a proliferation of white blood cells to get rid of the invader! This does not happen when we eat raw plant foods.

4.2
VEGAN NUTRITION

A low-fat, fruit-based alkalinizing, properly combined vegan diet is the only way to go for healing C&C and staying healthy. The author has never heard of a lasting healing of C&C by a non-vegan. Every essential nutrient needed for peak health, including the highest quality protein and all essential fatty acids, is available from plant foods and fruits (including avocados, nuts and seeds). Superior nutrition is food from the garden and orchard, unchanged by the heat of cooking. Cooked animal foods, oils and refined grains ruin our health. Cooked fats, oils and proteins are highly toxic, clogging and carcinogenic. Protein in cooked meat and pasteurized dairy foods has been rendered useless and toxic. As physician Dr. John McDougall puts it: "Pasteurized milk is nothing more than watery fat." Raw milk from cows and goats is not recommended either, due to its high fat content, allergenic and mucous-forming potential, inappropriate hormones and chemical residues from commercially-fed animals and because those with a history of C&C typically do not digest milk proteins well. Our optimal source of protein is from raw plant foods: nuts, seeds, fruits and vegetables. We can build as much muscle as we desire on a vegan diet after we have detoxified, healed and rejuvenated.

Although a change to a proper, nutritious diet (along with complete rest) is a key element in the wholistic care of persons with C&C, there is no standard plan for its implementation. Each advanced case must be evaluated via a thorough questionnaire and monitored individually. Changes must be made gradually and properly. Too rapid changes, such as the sudden addition of too much fruit or rough vegetables, can result in worsened gastric distress and increased elimination. Go slowly. If you are unsure about how to proceed, contact the author for a phone consultation.

Some people with C&C have mild symptoms of diarrhea or constipation, and some are debilitated with extensive inflammation, bloody diarrhea and spasms or constipation. Those with mild C&C or advanced C&C must avoid whole raw vegetables and transition to a vegan diet of soft non-acidic sweet fruits, steamed vegetables, squash and potatoes and fresh fruit and vegetable juices. Those with active inflammation need also to avoid nuts and seeds until they heal. The key to finding the right dietary plan is to work with an experienced professional health counselor, to tune in to the signals the body is sending and obey its higher intelligence.

With a change to a clean, energizing vegan diet, the body's intelligence system enacts a thorough housecleaning, whereby stored toxic matter is eliminated. This catabolic process of detoxification leads to weight loss in every case. Losing weight as one cleans out is often unsettling; however, this is the body's intelligent response to the toxemia and it is only temporary. The cleaner the body becomes, the faster it will heal. When the body is cleaned out and the belly is flat and thin, bodily energy and appetite will rise. Then, weight gain (or the anabolic rebuilding phase) will ensue. It takes time, diligence and patience to clean out, rebuild and rejuvenate. Many people have taken this road to health and are thankful they stayed with it. After a few years, if we live correctly, our body will have regenerated every cell, and youthful vitality with no more illness can be ours.

NOTE: During the healing diet transition phase, complete rest at home or at a Hygienic health care facility is recommended in all cases. People with active flare-ups who are working, caring for family members or are in school are advised to arrange to take a sabbatical and get complete rest until health is restored—the body requires rest to accomplish healing and typically cannot accomplish healing otherwise.

With those thoughts in mind, the following discussion on several key elements of nutritious eating should be used as a reference only. Their implementation requires intuitive wholistic thinking. Guidance from an experienced health counselor, such as the author, is advised.

Water

Taken in its pure form, water assists in the transport and elimination of toxins. Over time, water taken orally will also help loosen up stagnant food matter in the bowel. Those with chronic fatigue from C&C will also experience a rise in their energy level and a freshening effect with the increased use of pure water. Distilled or multi-filtered purified water is recommended. Self-purification of the body and healing occur as stored impurities are displaced by pure water. In the process, pure water increases the conductance of electrochemical nerve energy. The detoxifying effect of increased water use usually results in some discomfort as toxins are released from cells and tissues and eliminated. In cases of severe toxemia accompanying C&C, it is prudent to drink plenty of water.

Water fasting has proven to be a beneficial means of assisting the healing of C&C and the maintenance of health. There is at least one documented case history of a medical doctor who healed himself of colitis in this way. The definition of "fast" is a complete physiological rest (in bed), including abstinence from all food and nutriment except pure water. This enables the body to utilize virtually all available energy for self-healing; all activities are ceased and energy conserved for the organism to use for self-healing. Fasting is generally not necessary for recovery from C&C, however, it can be prudent and necessary in certain cases. Fasting must be undertaken only when conditions are favorable and not when severe malnutrition is present or when a person is unable to take complete rest; a Hygienic Doctor can make that determination. If you are interested in fasting, read Dr. Herbert M. Shelton's book *Fasting For Renewal of Life,* see Appendix C–Hygienic Health Care

Providers in this book and contact the author for a referral to a qualified professional fasting practitioner.

Fresh Air

Those with C&C who live in areas with polluted air will recover more easily in a location where the air is cleaner. Exercise is also very important as it ventilates the body, increasing circulation and oxygenation of the capillary system, which are vital factors for cellular repair. Stagnation of the capillary system is a primary factor in inflammatory disorders. Faster and more vigorous blood circulation promotes better capillary health due to greater oxygen uptake and rejuvenation of function.

Fruit

Raw fruits, excluding citrus fruits (which can bring on too rapid detoxification), are the ideal food for those seeking to recover from C&C. As revealed by studies of anthropology, biology and physiology, humans are frugivores. Thus, it is most healthful to include fresh raw fruits in the diet. However, some people who have been eating mostly cooked foods must gradually transition into a diet of plenty of fruit to avoid bringing on too rapid detoxification. Gradual diet changes are the safe way to proceed.

Fruit is the most naturally delicious and energizing food and is the perfect breakfast food. Fruit is the best source of caloric fuel for humans. In response to the question, "Where will I get my calories from on the Vegan Healing Diet?," the answer is: fruit. Fruits are abundant in sugars, which provide the best and, certainly, the most enjoyable source of caloric sustenance. Fruit is "nature's candy" and, not coincidentally, humans' most nutritious and sustaining food.

The healthiest, happiest, most energetic and bright-minded people known by the author thrive on a fruit-based diet. Ripe fruits are naturally appealing, non-mucous forming, predigested (thus requiring little digestive energy), high in sun-drenched water and are most nourishing and energizing. The nutrients in ripe fruits include sugars, proteins, hormones, enzymes, vitamins, minerals and pure water. The skins of fruits contain "friendly" bacteria. Tough skins, such as those on apples, should be removed while recovering from C&C. Most fruits contain fiber, and the ones which do not, such as papaya, do not cause constipation due to their high water content, enzymes and stimulating sugars. Digested fruit leaves behind little residue, which is most beneficial for C&C. All watery fruits are valuable for their cleansing properties. Sweet fruits contain pectin, which helps bind stools. Ripe bananas, papayas, peeled apples, pears, grapes, mangos, dates and melons have given C&C sufferers the best healing results. Ripe bananas stand out as the best of all foods for promoting healing of C&C and restoring the formation of stools; they may be eaten as the predominant food during and after the healing phase.

Because fruits require very short retention time in the stomach, they must always be eaten alone, on an empty stomach, in order to prevent fermentation. Fruit should not be eaten within six hours after eating cooked food, or better yet, wait until the next day's breakfast. If fermentation results even when following those guidelines, this may indicate that the stomach is not clean. In that case, the drinking of water to cleanse the stomach upon arising is beneficial. It is best to eat fruit and only fruit as the first meal of the day, whole or juiced, because when we eat heavier foods our morning detoxification is suspended. In the morning persons with C&C may find that their systems cannot handle foods heavier than fruit. As previously stated, a transition to a fruit-based diet should be made gradually; too rapid a transition can bring on many problems. The author is an expert diet counselor and is available to assist. Living Nutrition magazine contains many helpful articles by the world's premier educators and doctors on fruit eating and natural lifestyle.

Dr. T. C. Fry wrote the following article regarding human's natural dietetic character:

Are We Frugivores?

First, some outstanding facts for your consideration:

1. While in a state of nature, humans and, as well, other species developed natural equipment and faculties for finding, taking, consuming, efficiently processing and utilizing foods to which they adapted.

2, Despite the many and varied diets consumed by humans over the globe, our instinctual dietary nature and faculties have not evolved away from our pristine foods.

3. The foods upon which we developed in nature necessarily nourished us adequately to bring us to our high state of development. The foods to which we adapted in nature will still sustain us adequately and amply by meeting all our varied nutrient requirements.

4. With our modern botanical and horticultural expertise, we are capable of producing our natural foods of a quality that will continue to meet our nutrient needs and enable us to attain our highest potentials.

5. Symbiosis and cooperation exist in nature to an extent we do not realize. Certainly our educational media and texts do not teach our symbiotic role in nature. Humans existed symbiotically in nature.

Are we a species of fruit-eaters? Would you, in nature, relish ripe grapes, peaches, melons, bananas, apples, plums, oranges, mangos, avocados, tomatoes, figs, berries and the thousands of other fruits? Would fruits attract your eye, tantalize your sense of smell, and be a gustatory delight in their raw natural ripe state? Would you prefer anything that occurs in nature to a juicy, sweet watermelon?

Man has always had a love affair going with fruits. Even through all his perversions, he has continued to relish fruits. Fruits are the natural food of humans and the only food category ideally suited to all their faculties. This does not mean we should eat fruits totally and exclusively in our present circumstances, but it does mean that, in nature, that's all we ate as attested to by anthropological evidence scientists have uncovered, notably Dr. Alan Walker of Johns Hopkins University.

Of course, you go for fruits in their raw state regardless of what else your acculturation and circumstances dispose you to eat. Your instincts are still alive and well despite perversions. Many myths have been built around and about fruits.

Nutritionists, so-called, are the creatures of training dictated by the meat, grain and milk trusts. These trusts are part of the dominant commercial interests that dictate what will be taught in our educational institutions from universities down to kindergarten. Nutritionists are trained like seals to parrot the propaganda which will induce the populace to consume their masters' products, with the basic five food groups being one of the primary propaganda weapons put at their disposal to serve their masters. Of course, there are renegade nutritionists and dietitians who have revolted against the basic four except for the fruit and vegetable category. Most nutritionists are ashamed of the fifth food category and don't even mention it though it is on the books along with the basic four.

The fifth category consists of what might broadly be termed "accessory foods" such as oils, syrups, snack foods, sugars, wines, seasonings, jams, preserves, etc. Even though we are admonished to eat from all five food categories daily by the framers of this scheme to peddle commercial products, nutritionists and dietitians are not keen on mouthing this part of the propaganda even though they include it liberally in their recipes.

While some nutritionists and dietitians praise fruits and vegetables, they still characterize those who point out our biologically correct foods as faddists and nutritional quacks. Yet, even in seminars, those who sharply question me must admit that, aesthetically, they would eat little besides fruits in nature and that we humans are naturally fruitarians.

All the criteria heretofore cited as the requirements of our natural foods are amply met by fruits. In short, they are replete with our nutrient requirements in practically the proportions that we need them.

Dr. Bruce Ames of the University of California, Berkeley, has created a catalog of poisons in vegetables and published an extensive article in the September 23, 1983 issue of Science *magazine. No indictment of fruits as having toxic substances was made or can be made. Virtually every vegetable was indicted. All were a part of the same study. Humans are biologically equipped to handle most fruits.*

When ripened, fruits accommodatingly convert their carbohydrate components into glucose and fructose, simple sugars we can use without further digestion. Their enzymes convert their proteins into amino acids and their fats into fatty acids and glycerols. Thus, when we eat fruits, all we need do is savor their goodness. The fruit portions, that is, mesocarps, were specifically compounded to attract biological symbionts. Fruits meet their nutrient needs rather ideally with predigested nutrients. For humans, no other food compares with fruits in satisfying all needs including, of course, our requirement for delicious soul-exalting fare.

I'm sure that you will agree through your own senses that fruits would be your primary food in a state of nature.

Fruits really have it all; all that it took to make us into superb human beings; all that is required to sustain us in a healthy state insofar as food contributes to this condition; and all that we need to live a long, rewarding and happy life.

Does fruit have too much sugar? Dried fruit certainly contains concentrated sugar and should be soaked or ingested with some water. However, fresh ripe fruits contain 80% to 95% water and are, therefore, not too sugary. Each of our cells' only fuel source is sugar. That is only one reason why sweet fruits should be eaten as the main food in our diet. Dr. T. C. Fry wrote the following article to address the charge that fruits have too much sugar:

Obviously this charge is made by those who have not weighed or cogitated upon the considerations. Or those who refuse to recognize the evidence. First, about 90% of our nutrient requirements aside from water are for monosaccharides (simple sugars are glucose, fructose, glycerose and galactose) for energy. Until you've met this need, it is ridiculous to cry "too much sugar." Sugar in fruits comes to us predigested, hence it can't be beyond our digestive capacity, though it may go on down the intestinal tube if ingested beyond absorptive capacity which, too, is unlikely because of the satiety factor which limits fruit-eating to actual replenishment needs.

Fruit sugars are said to be absorbed "too fast," but they do not present nearly the problem with their fructose content as digested starches which are all glucose. Recent research has proven that the glucose (rated at 100 as a sugar load factor) of starches (mostly grains and tubers in our case) is absorbed just as fast as fruit sugars. Moreover, they "storm" the body's sugar metabolizing faculties more greatly than do fruit sugars, with the component fructose (rated at 29 as a sugar load factor). If we eat "too much sugar," that is, caloric values exceeding our needs, then obviously we've overeaten. In the case of sugar, the surplus is either stored as fats or harmlessly excreted.

Let's look at starches, often called complex carbohydrates. These must be heated to be broken down from long chain polysaccharides or starch. Heating dextrinizes starches. However, because there are no immediate sugars to absorb for appestat control, overeating of dextrinized starches is endemic. And many athletes intentionally eat heavily of starchy foods (dextrinized by heat) as in "carbohydrate loading." As dextrinized starches are converted to glucose, once absorption starts, according to recent research, our bloodstream is hit with as big a sugar load as fruits present!

As to excess sugar, we're more likely to get it from starches which we're more likely to overeat than from fruits which quickly satisfy the appestat. In the case of heated starches, unless heated at very low temperatures for an extended period of time, our fungal and bacterial flora can readily ferment it, thus intoxicating us to some extent. Uncooked sugars are not fermentable until they have been oxidized, a process unlikely to happen with these quickly absorbed foods unless other factors delay their absorption. When explored and examined, the charge of "excessive sugar" vanishes.

As a last consideration, fruits are alkaline in their metabolic end-products. The body readily excretes excess alkalis whereas it must neutralize objectionable acids and excrete them if capable. (Arthritis, bursitis, rheumatism, gout and yet other problems are caused by the body's inability to excrete base salts from acid neutralization, usually calcium salts. For instance the uric acid of meats are neutralized into calcium urate crystals because we do not secrete the enzyme uricase as carnivores do. These salts have an affinity for cartilage in joints. Also having this affinity are the acid end products of grains, oxalic acids in vegetables like spinach, chard, beets and lamb's-quarter, most cooked foods, and meats.)

Dr. T. C. Fry wrote the following article on humans' natural relationship with fruit:

Humans and Fruit: Symbiotic Partners In Life

While few biology books proclaim symbiosis and none that I've encountered proclaim our own symbiotic role in nature, we are symbionts as are thousands of species. Symbiosis is cooperation between dissimilar organisms for mutual benefit. Symbionts are cooperators in symbiotic living. While the word "symbiont" is supposed to apply only to the lesser of two cooperating organisms, I prefer to call both of the complementary cooperators symbionts for that is the only nomenclature that makes sense. Let us observe this phenomenon in nature.

We see flowers bloom and put forth tons upon tons of pollen for fertilizing the ovaries of female flowers. Both male and female flowers secrete nectar at their inner base to attract consumption by bees and other insects. In taking such a large reward, the bees and insects become contaminated with pollen in the male flowers only to have it removed when they take the nectar of female flowers. The ovaries of female flowers secrete a sticky substance which the bee or insect must come in contact with in taking their nectars. Instances of symbiosis abound in nature.

The above is cited to demonstrate natural cooperativeness or symbiosis. In this case, we see that the flowers of plants, both woody and non-woody, attracted bees and insects to take the free meals provided. This is the way that plants uncannily solved the problem of fertilization, attesting to a high order of intelligence in plant life (which is perceived by few).

Humans do not collect nectar. Even if they did, it would be a very poor food though it sustains bees and other insects well. Fertilization in this manner is necessary to certain forms of plant life to insure that seeds be created with which to propagate the species. As we know, plant life is stationary. Once it has created its seed progeny, a new problem arises, that of scattering the seeds so they will flourish. How did this uncanny wisdom in nature accomplish this?

Among the many solutions was that of creating yet another food around the seed or seeds. In attracting consumption of this food by mobile creatures, there was the incidental distribution of its seeds to areas where they would not compete for space and raw materials with the parent plant. Of course, that same immense wisdom dictated the creation of seeds that were unappetizing so they would be discarded rather than consumed.

But the greatest wisdom of all, perhaps, was that which created the food package to proportionately meet the precise needs of its eaters: those creatures which, in taking and becoming dependent on these foods, became the fruit plant's biological symbiont. That this method of seed distribution was successful is evidenced by the thousands of kinds of fruits created around seeds in nature. Fruits attract human senses in nature and are gourmet delights in their natural ripened state, which ensures their survival. Also, fruits contain no poisons in the fresh ripened state whereas almost all plants and seeds contain components which we cannot metabolize, hence are toxic directly or indirectly.

Fruits in nature are in a predigested form when they ripen. They are beautiful to behold and emit captivating aromas and fragrances. This makes them irresistibly attractive to their biological symbionts. If all the water and fiber is removed from most of these fruits, the predigested carbohydrates are almost all the same, about 350 calories per 100 grams on average, more than enough to meet the energy needs of biological symbionts. This is about 88% of solids.

In like manner, fruits supply from 4 to 8 grams of amino acids per 100 grams, almost every one of them with all the essential amino acids in about the proportions that humans require, plus, of course, other amino acids. The average amino acid content is about the same as mother's milk for a growing baby. The average is about 6% of solids. When sufficient calories have been consumed to meet caloric needs, intake is almost double our actual daily amino acid shortfall from recycling.

Further, the fatty acids from almost all fruits other than avocados and olives constitute about 1% to 5% of solids other than fiber. These fatty acids are liberal in their supply of the essential fatty acids. The average fatty acid content of fruits is about 2%.

But, importantly, fruits are rich in mineral matter in the most utilizable form in all nature! Of its solids, about 3% are minerals including, of course, ample calcium to meet our needs if we do not eat more than 20% acid-forming foods and if we do not cook and derange fruit nutrients.

Of the labeled macronutrients, there are vitamins which are really micronutri-

ents, so little as not to be ordinarily measurable. A year of the RDAs for vitamins would not fill a sewing thimble! Yet, fruits supply many multiples of the RDAs of vitamins in almost every instance. For instance, vitamin C in fruits sufficient to meet our caloric needs is about ten times as much, on average, as the RDA for it.

As humans developed exclusively on fruits, they failed to develop water drinking faculties. Those on the fruit diet have 60% to 70% less need for water than those on the conventional diet, primarily because pathogens require inordinate amounts of water to hold them in suspension and carry them out of the body. Fruits supply ample water in its purest form to meet our needs. Fruitarians do not normally drink water, but make as many trips to the urinal as anyone.

We are biological symbionts of fruit-bearing plants and in nature would eat very little besides fruits. Despite all this, there's no particular harm in eating green leafy vegetables, stalks, stems and their fresh juices in the raw state. Even some steaming or conservative cooking of tubers, stalks, stems, roots, corns and selected legumes and grains (preferably sprouted) are not sufficiently deleterious to seriously harm our health. Of course, there are some toxic results from eating all this cooked fare and we're better off without it. Yet, I repeat, there is no great harm in their consumption relative to what is suffered from conventional fare.

Vegetables, Squash and Potatoes

Well-grown vegetables, squash and potatoes are rich in nutrients and generally have more fiber and minerals than fruits. For their nourishing properties, steamed vegetables and fresh-made raw-living juices are highly recommended for self-healing C&C. Raw vegetables are more nourishing than cooked vegetables, which have had their life force, enzymes and vitamins degraded or destroyed by heat; however, lightly steamed vegetables (as well as squash and potatoes) are still very nourishing and are recommended. Again, raw vegetables and salads are NOT recommended for people with C&C flare-ups or active inflammation—they can irritate the bowel, so it is best to juice them and steam them during the healing phase.

Vegetables, squash and potatoes supply valuable mineral salts. Minerals act as cofactors for our digestive enzymes, making them more effective. Minerals also serve as cofactors for our cellular enzymes, assisting in the conversion of nutrients into fuel and in the offloading of toxins. Without a regular supply of these cofactors, health cannot be maintained.

People who have overcome C&C need to focus on thorough mastication when eating whole vegetables in order to reduce the digestive responsibilities of the stomach and small intestine. Blended vegetable salads (made in a blender or food processor with some water or fresh vegetable juice) are recommended for those with weak digestion. Irritating vegetables, such as onions, radishes and garlic (actually an herb), must be avoided. As one begins eating a more and more natural diet, a natural appreciation for vegetables will be gained. And with this, one will no longer need to use flavorings and irritating condiments, which mask the true flavor of foods and impair the body's ability to sense their digestive enzyme requirements.

Vitamins

Vitamin deficiency typically plays a major role in the development of C&C. The role of vitamins becomes even more crucial during the manifestation of C&C because of the accelerated loss of body tissue and fluids stemming from the ravaging effects of inflammation, the body's resorting to the use of its nutrient stores, and increased elimination.

All of the vitamins essential for robust health can be obtained by eating a diet of fruits, vegetables, seeds and nuts grown in healthy soil. We also need daily sunshine in order to make our own vitamin D. Some vitamins, including some B's and K, are made in the gut, as long as there are healthy flora. However, there is controversy as to whether we actually utilize those vitamins. Flora imbalances brought on by malnutrition, frequent bowel movements, drugs, enemas and colonics can inhibit the manufacture of these vitamins. Vitamins from fresh plant and fruit foods and the sun are our perfect sources; vitamin pills are to varying degrees toxic, unusable and not recommended. The following is a discussion of the vitamins which are key in nutritional healing for C&C:

A

Also called carotene, A's absorption may be impaired with C&C. Carotene in plants is converted to A in the liver. A is needed for the repair of mucous membranes. The best natural sources of A are green and yellow vegetables and yellow fruits. Carrots and carrot juice are high in carotene.

B Complex

All of the B vitamins are needed to nourish the nervous system, assist in energy management, repair tissue and facilitate digestion. All are available from whole plant and fruit foods, including vitamin B_{12} which is also manufactured in our gut by bacteria. Under normal conditions, vitamin B_{12} need not be obtained from animal sources or supplements or shots. However, if there is a critically-low level, as confirmed by a urinary methylmalonic acid (uMMA) test (the only reliable test for vitamin B_{12}), methylcobalamin (vitamin B_{12}) supplements or shots are recommended. Vitamin B_{12} absorption requires a certain polypeptide called "intrinsic factor" which is produced by the parietal cells of the stomach. In cases of malnutrition and intestinal inflammation, intrinsic factor may not be produced and absorption of all vitamins will be impaired. B vitamins are destroyed by sulfa drugs. For more information on vitamin B_{12}, refer to the following section.

C

Also called ascorbic acid, C is necessary for improving the adsorption of iron, repairing blood vessels and mucous membranes. The best natural sources are raw bell peppers and citrus fruits. C supplementation is not recommended—overdosage results in loose stools.

D

The "sunshine vitamin," D helps with the assimilation of vitamin A, nerve function, blood clotting and combats depression. The best sources are sunshine (at least 15 minutes in the sun each day), sunflower seeds and nuts.

E

Also called tochopherol, E is an antioxidant which is important in preventing the oxidation of fats. E also helps maintain healthy blood vessels and muscles. Best natural sources are leafy greens.

K

Also called menadione, K helps prevent internal bleeding and hemorrhages. Some sources list vitamin K deficiency as a cause of colitis. K can be formed by bacteria in the gut. K's best natural sources are green leafy, cruciferous and sea vegetables. X-rays and aspirin destroy vitamin K.

P

Also called bioflavinoids, P is necessary for the healthy function of the mucous membranes, capillaries and immune function. Some nutrition books list vitamin P deficiency as a source of colitis. P's best natural sources are citrus fruits, cherries and grapes.

U

Little is known about vitamin U, but it is thought to play a role in helping the body heal bowel ulcerations. U is found in raw cabbage juice. Since cabbage juice is high in sulfur, which can be irritating to the bowel, the intake of this juice should be minimized.

Minerals

Numerous studies have shown that minerals are a major determinant in our health and a broad spectrum, including the trace minerals, is essential for excellent health and longevity. Modern agricultural methods rely on only a few basic mineral compounds in their fertilizer and the soils they grow in are largely depleted in trace minerals. Even organic agriculture may not produce mineral-rich produce since many areas are deficient in trace minerals. Only recently have some organic growers begun to recognize the benefits of spreading rock powder amendments (also called rock dust) on their soils. Rock powder is derived from glacial or volcanic deposits and contains a broad spectrum of mineral elements (typically, over 90).

Because people with C&C typically become deficient in many minerals, they will benefit from eating as much high-mineral-content food as possible. The best natural food sources of minerals are vegetables and fruits. These foods contain the mineral salts we need in health-promoting organic, electrolyte form. That is, the minerals are chelated, or bound to organic molecules, in ionic solution, as required by the body. In this form the minerals are nontoxic. Ionic and crystalline salts from sea water and land deposits are also rich in minerals but they are not chelated and, thus, they are toxic—one or two ounces of solid salt taken at once is deadly. While they can be used in emergency situations when there is critically low mineral or electrolyte level, they are not health-promoting, they contain many toxic elements and they should be avoided. Salt users who have C&C only heal after they discontinue salt use and adopt the diet program described herein.

Mineral supplements derived from rock powders are poorly used and can cause many problems, including deposits in joints, arterial plaque and metabolic and neurological imbalances. Furthermore, these are not recognized as food by the body and the body will attempt to excrete them, wasting your precious energy and money. Therefore, mineral supplements are not recommended because the body needs a full spectrum of organically-bound (naturally chelated) minerals as provided by nature in whole fresh plant foods.

Vegetables are the densest source of minerals. Freshly made vegetable juices are very useful for remineralizing the body. Minerals (and other nutrients) are released from the fibers of vegetables by mechanical juicers far more efficiently than by the masticating action of our teeth. Celery juice is the richest food source of electrolytes (especially organic sodium salts) and a most healthful source of minerals for those needing to make up severe mineral deficiencies.

Sea vegetables are the richest food source of minerals. Sea vegetables must be soaked and thoroughly rinsed to remove as much sea salt as possible. Only the softest varieties, such as dulse, in raw, whole leaf form, are recommended. Some varieties are too fibrous and tough for our teeth and digestive juices to break down and release the minerals. The use of sea vegetables is not recommended during the healing phase of C&C because they are too fibrous.

Green vegetable and grass and plant powders are rich in many minerals. They can be beneficial when obtained in organic, low-temperature-processed form and added to fresh juices. Barley powder is mild while wheatgrass powder has a stronger flavor which is too intense for most people. Products which are free of additives are best. For people in the throes of a severe detox, these powders are not recommended as they can accelerate the symptoms.

Blue-green micro-algaes in powder, flake and liquid form (spirulina, super blue-green, etc.) are also rich in a broad spectrum of minerals and other nutrients. However, they are not recommended for many reasons, including: 1. they are extremely concentrated sources of protein, which tends to putrefy in the bowel; 2. they are overstimulating, imparting a false sense of "feeling better" while enervating our organism; 3. some are cultivated in tanks with salt water which imparts a salty residue; 4. some are dried at high temperatures, damaging and altering the nutrients; and 5. all contain phycocyanin, a bitter protoplasmic poison.

"Superfood" is a new term for a variety of concentrated nutrient products. None are recommended; they are too stimulating and unbalancing and their use is conducive to disordered eating.

The following is a discussion of the minerals which are key in nutritional healing for C&C. Studies have found that most of these are deficient in persons with C&C. Here are the key minerals which are needed in relation to bowel health for nerve and muscle repair and function:

Calcium

Calcium is very important in nerve function and the contraction of muscles, including the intestines. Some sources list calcium deficiency as a factor in colitis. Relief from bowel cramping may be alleviated by eating calcium-rich foods. Calcium is also important in hormone secretion and blood clotting, and it may help prevent cancer in cases of C&C. For calcium to be absorbed efficiently, the wall of the small intestine needs to be clean and a healthy population of flora must be present. The body's metabolism of calcium depends upon the presence of sufficient magnesium. The best natural sources of calcium are most vegetables including soft, thoroughly-rinsed sea vegetables (such as whole leaf dulse), plus fruits, seeds and nuts.

Magnesium

Magnesium is also very important in muscle and nerve function, making it another key nutrient in relaxing bowel cramping and spasms and improving bowel motion. It is also important in blood sugar metabolism and the function of protein. Magnesium is a cofactor in about 300 of the body's enzymes, so it helps our cells assimilate nutrients and expel wastes. It also has an alkalinizing effect on the body's fluids. Its best natural sources are nuts, dark green and root vegetables, figs, citrus fruits, apples and sea vegetables.

Potassium

Potassium is beneficial for soothing nerves and muscle cramps, relieving diarrhea and transporting wastes for elimination. It is plentiful in bananas, nuts, avocados and many other fruits and vegetables.

Sodium

Sodium helps keep the nerves and muscles functioning properly and works to keep calcium and other minerals soluble in the blood. Sodium deficiency is cited as a factor in digestion problems. Its best natural sources are carrots, celery, beets and artichokes. Celery juice is high in sodium. (Avoid crystalline salt—it is toxic.)

Here are four key minerals which are needed for blood sugar metabolism, which is typically disordered in cases of C&C:

Zinc

Zinc is a critical cofactor with many enzymes, is essential for protein synthesis and ulcer healing, muscle contraction, helps maintain the body's acid-alkaline balance, enhances immune function and protects against fatigue and depression. Its best natural sources are pumpkin seeds, nuts and root vegetables.

Manganese

Manganese is important in insulin production and, possibly, thyroid hormone production and is a cofactor for many enzymes. It also helps eliminate fatigue and improves muscle reflexes. Its best natural sources are green leafy vegetables, nuts, seeds and blueberries.

Chromium

Chromium is a trace mineral used in the metabolism of sugar which may help alleviate irritability associated with hypoglycemia, a condition which can be related to digestive disorders and C&C. The best natural sources are beets and walnuts. Walnuts should only be eaten fresh within a short time of the fall harvest as they go rancid quickly.

Iodine

Iodine is important in the function of the thyroid, which controls metabolism. It helps relieve irritability and nervousness, symptoms that go hand in hand with C&C. Its best availability is in sea vegetables. The most easily digested sea vegetable is dulse (which is very soft). Whole leaf dulse must be soaked and rinsed in pure water; then, the moisture can be squeezed out by hand before eating. Sea vegetables can be eaten plain, in salads, or blended in vegetable juices.

Iron

Iron is essential in the building of healthy blood, which works to overcome fatigue and anemia. Its best natural sources are seeds, nuts, green leafy vegetables, asparagus, beets, avocados, watermelon, peaches, apricots, grapes, dates and raisins.

Selenium

Selenium is a trace mineral which works with vitamin E as an antioxidant, counteracting environmental pollutants. It is also an immune enhancer. It may also work against colon cancer. Its best natural sources are nuts, broccoli and tomatoes.

Silicon

Silicon is important in the formation of resilient connective tissue in organs and blood vessels and possibly helps deliver light energy into the cells. It is abundant in cucumbers, green leafy vegetables and beets.

Protein

Protein is one of the two largest dietary concerns (the other being the suitability of fruit) which arise for people considering this vegan diet approach. Concerns and fears are typically rooted in common erroneous beliefs: social conditioning which is based on falsehoods about health and nutrition stemming from at least a century of propaganda propagated by the meat, dairy and medical industries.

The happy truth about protein is that even the simplest vegan diet is an abundantly sufficient source of superior protein (actually, the building blocks of protein, from which all animals build their protein: amino acids) and we don't have to worry about it except in extreme cases of emaciation. High-protein foods cause virtually all cases of C&C and they are not needed, not even digestible and only serve to exacerbate C&C. Fruits and vegetables are premium, sufficient sources of amino acids, the building blocks of protein which our cells (primarily those of the liver) use to synthesize ALL of its protein. No—the protein in the flesh and muscles of a meat eater and milk drinker is not comprised of the very protein molecules which were ingested. Rather, that protein was synthesized from the amino acids which were reduced from protein molecules and assimilated after digestion in the small intestine.

Another happy truth is that the body recycles approximately 80% of the protein it makes. As such, we do not need to concern ourselves with eating an abundance of protein every day because we simply do not normally lose much.

Those who believe that they are deriving quality protein from cooked meats are mistaken. The protein from cooked foods is largely destroyed or rendered unusable by the heat. In actuality, very little protein or amino acids are available from meat and dairy or any other cooked foods. Then how is it possible to grow and build muscle if little protein is available from meat and dairy?

All our protein needs are provided by plants and their fruits. Synthesis of the eight essential amino acids occurs in plants, but not in humans. Only plants extract nitrogen from the air and nitrates from the soil for amino acid synthesis. Humans and other animals obtain essential amino acids from plant foods, including fruits. Plants and fruits would not exist without amino acids as part of their structures. The nonessential amino acids are synthesized within our bodies by digestive reduction of more complex amino acids (protein molecules) into simpler amino acids.

A broad diet of plant foods which excludes any and all animal foods provides all eight essential amino acids required by the body for all its protein needs. We will get enough amino acids if we simply eat vegan meals of appropriate foods in quantities which are satisfying. Countless vegans, including people who've successfully healed C&C and adopted the vegan lifestyle, have found their new eating style to be more satisfying and beneficial than their previous meat-based diets.

The following article appeared in *Living Nutrition vol. 19.*

Protein Facts and Fallacies

by Dr. Douglas Graham

Although protein was the first nutrient to be discovered and named, most people are still worried about getting enough. This is paradoxical, as protein shortage is a practically unknown condition. Even though we learned in grammar school Biology that the nucleus of every living cell contains DNA, which is made of protein, many people still think that foods such as fruits and vegetables are devoid of protein. This in spite of the fact that these same people know full well that there are many species of creatures in nature that live out their life span eating nothing but fruits and veggies.

We don't really need to crunch a great many numbers in order to determine our true protein needs. Protein is an essential building block for growth; human mother's milk averages about 7% of its calories from protein. This enables an infant to grow at meteoric speed while gaining as much as 12 pounds in just 6 months. It can be safely assumed that adults need no more protein per calorie than an infant, as the adult's growth rate is far slower. Various types of research and countless studies have confirmed that mid-single digit protein consumption, as a function of total calories consumed, is more than enough for our requirements.

Health seekers have tested this concept fully through the use of fasting as a method of healing from injury and disease. While following a "diet" of rest and water, sometimes for 30 to 40 days or even longer, protein deficiency has never been encountered in fasters. The body demonstrated that it had sufficient protein available by successfully working its healing magic during the fasts.

A wide variety of bodily ills are overcome during water fasts, including those that definitely require protein, such as wound and bone healing. This shows that humans carry a large protein reserve of what are called "labile proteins," ones that are not structurally integrated. Therefore, heavy protein consumption is not necessary on a daily basis. In fact, the overconsumption of dense protein source foods typically results in harm to one's health.

The Problem With High Protein Foods

Fruits and vegetables have long been considered health foods. A diet consisting of nothing but fruits and vegetables will supply a protein content of about 8% per calorie. It has been shown repeatedly that diets supplying double digit protein per calorie consumed leads to a variety of health problems including heart and vascular disease, kidney disorders, liver dysfunction, arthritis and a wide variety of cancers.

A primary reason for these problems is foods that are rich in protein are usually also very high in fat. It is rare to find a high protein food that does not have fat as its primary source of calories. Certainly this is true of all flesh foods, dairy, nuts and seeds.

Whole Food Nutrition or Fragmented Nutrition?

Empty calorie foods, or "junk foods," are defined as calorie sources sans full nutrient content. Refined calorie sources, whether they are protein, fat, or carbohydrates, supply empty calories. We generally think of sugar and empty calories as being synonymous. Refined starches (e.g., flour products) also qualify as empty calories, even though the general public may think of them as "healthy carbs." Refined oils, too, must be recognized as empty calorie foods, since they are neither whole foods nor do they provide the full complement of nutrients found in the original source. Of course, protein powders of all types also qualify as empty calories as they fit the definition perfectly. It is sometimes difficult to accept that our beloved supplements are no more than junk foods. Nevertheless, flax or any other oil, hemp or any other protein powder, white flour and refined sugar all fall into the same category: empty calories. When you add any of them to your fruits and vegetables, you turn health food into junk food.

Rather than ask, "Where do you get your protein?", consumers of such refined, isolated empty calories should be asking, "Where do you get your nutrients?" Protein from a can is no more nutritious than sugar from a bag or oil from a bottle; all of these items qualify as junk when compared to whole foods.

Protein Does Not Build Muscle

Some may argue that we need to eat great volumes of protein in order to build muscle mass. In fact, if we wish to be able to exercise with sufficient intensity to spur growth in our muscles and related structures, we need to consume sufficient carbohydrates to meet our fuel needs—preferably from fruit.

Since protein is one of the three caloronutrients (along with carbohydrates and fats), protein fuel demands rise only when one's diet is deficient in carbohydrates (as the body is forced to convert the protein into carbohydrates—a very inefficient, energy-draining process).

Eating protein does not build muscle. Muscular growth results from placing a strength overload upon the muscles and then supplying adequate conditions for recovery. Repeatedly using this overload and recovery strategy results in steady and reliable muscular growth and development. The quality of tissue developed will be determined by the foods eaten, and the highest quality tissues will develop as a result of eating fruits and vegetables.

Protein, per se, is not actually used by the body to build new tissue. When foods are eaten, their constituent proteins are broken down during the digestive processes into ever smaller particles: proteoles, polypeptides, dipeptides, and, eventually, amino acids. The amino acids travel to the liver where they are recombined and constructed into the specific proteins needed at any given time.

Not only is it a fallacy that protein will result in muscle growth, but the concept that the body needs specific proteins, from fish, meat, eggs, etc. is also fallacious. The body breaks down all proteins to their component amino acids before recombining them. Eating the muscles from animals will not result in our developing bigger muscles. As an analogy, eating animals' eyes will not improve our vision, nor will eating their brains increase our intellect.

Whole Fruits and Vegetables Have All of the Protein We Need!

The protein content of fruits and vegetables is perfect for human beings, as it is for all of the animals in the anthropoid family. Gorillas have no trouble growing big and strong on fruits and veggies, and the same applies to us. Don't fall for yet another health-destroying gimmick. Eat fruits and veggies with confidence, knowing that you are supplying yourself with the world's most nutritious foods.

Fats and Oils

Fats and oils are essential to the human diet and may be obtained in sufficient quantities from whole plant sources. Fats and oils are needed for energy, cell membrane elasticity, hormone synthesis, insulation and many other functions.

During the healing phase, fatty foods must be eliminated from the diet and avoided until healing is complete. The body cannot digest these foods while we are ailing. Ingesting them will perpetuate or exacerbate inflammation and distress. They include: meats, dairy (milk, cream, cheese, yogurt, eggs), oils, avocados, nuts, seeds, coconuts and olives.

People who have healed from C&C have difficulty digesting fats in quantities they were accustomed to and are, therefore, advised to maintain a low-fat diet. Ripe fruits and fresh vegetable juices are easily digested and a sufficient source of fatty acids in the diet during the healing phase of C&C. Leafy green vegetables are an excellent source of fatty acids. It is not necessary to obtain all of the omega fatty acids; a variety of raw fruits and vegetables will sufficiently satisfy all of our fat needs.

During the post-healing phase, when heavier fatty/oily foods are desired, the best choice is avocado. Avocados are the best choice for satisfying cravings when transitioning off meat. As they are a tree-ripened fruit, avocados contain no cholesterol and abundantly healthful, easy-to-digest fatty acids (19 in all, including omegas 3 and 6). In some cases, it is best to slowly increase the amount of avocado in the diet, starting with an occasional slice. Others can eat and digest one whole avocado at a time. It is not recommended that whole avocados be eaten more than three times per week, nor in quantities exceeding one-half of an avocado per meal.

These foods can also be beneficial in small quantities during the post-healing phase: raw, whole soaked seeds and nuts, seed and nut butters and milks, and seed "cheese" (made by processing soaked and sprouted seeds). Fats and oils digest best when eaten with vegetables. It is not advisable to eat raw or sprouted nuts and seeds when intestinal or colon inflammation is present as they are difficult to digest and often contribute to toxemia and perpetuate inflammation.

Juicing

The drinking of fresh raw fruit and vegetable juices is highly recommended for persons with C&C. Juice therapy has been known to greatly improve chronic digestive troubles, help overcome ulcers, increase vitality and resolve many more health problems. There are many books available on juicing and many types of juicers at a wide range of prices. The author found his juicer to be worth its weight in gold during the early stages of his recovery. Juicers break open the cells of the vegetables or fruits, releasing minerals many times more effectively than our chewing can. Raw juices are rich in "organic" water, enzymes, vitamins and minerals, all of which assimilate within minutes.

Juices are best digested when slowly sipped and swished around in the mouth for mixing with digestive enzyme secretions. Several glasses of fresh juice may be used each day. Delicious "smoothies" may be made by blending juice with dates and/or fresh or frozen strawberries or bananas. Such drinks provide excellent nourishment for those who are having difficulty with solid foods.

Raw juices can promote fast detoxification, which needs to be regulated in some cases. A blender can also be used to liquefy fruits and vegetables so that all of the pulp is used. Blends of ripe bananas and water are excellent.

It is deliciously fun to experiment with fruit juices, of singular fruit or combinations. They include apple, pear, grape, apple-pear, apple-celery, grape-celery, pear-celery and many others. Vegetable juices recommended for C&C include carrot (contains vitamins B, C, D, E, G and K, plus many minerals), carrot-kale, carrot-cucumber, carrot-celery and carrot-cabbage. Wheat grass juice, which requires a special juicer, is very rich in nutrients; however, it is an aggressive detoxifier, typically unpleasant to the senses and not recommended. Those who desire to try wheat grass juice and find it too strong may try diluting it in carrot or orange juice.

Citrus juices are also beneficial for their nourishing and cleansing properties. However, citrus juices are not advisable for those with C&C because they typically trigger an acceleration in the body's detoxification response. Also, the citric acids typically irritate a sensitive, inflamed gut. After C&C is healed up, moderate amounts of sweet citrus juices can be used regularly by those following a proper health program.

Lactobacteria

Lactobacillus acidophilus, or "friendly bacteria," live symbiotically in the colon, working to keep it clean and to synthesize some vitamins. In most cases a healthy colon flora can be established soon after commencing the Vegan Diet recommended herein. Some people with C&C may not easily be able to establish a healthy flora, especially those who recently used antibiotics. There are various acidophilus/intestinal flora products available at healthfood stores with which you may experiment. Those powdered ones which are cultured in a vegan food base may help to improve stool formation as well as vitamin synthesis. Long-term use of such products is unnecessary.

Raw, salt-free sauerkraut is the most natural and potentially most effective way to supplement our bowel flora; however, it is typically not needed (but it may be most helpful after antibiotic use). Salted sauerkraut is unhealthful and should be avoided. While raw, salt-free sauerkraut is not commonly sold in healthfood stores, it can easily be made at home, as such: Blend the juice and pulp from approximately one-half of a freshly-juiced white cabbage with a few ounces of purified water as desired. Optionally, small amounts of finely chopped dill and/or fresh lemon or orange juice may be added to the sauerkraut for flavor. Store the sauerkraut blend in a loosely covered jar for three to seven days at room temperature then refrigerate it. Three days after its preparation, a small amount of the sauerkraut pulp or strained juice may be taken along with a glass of vegetable juice or with a dinner meal of vegetables, sweet potatoes and squash. Do not eat sauerkraut before, with or soon after any sweet fruit meals—the bacteria cultures will react with the fruit sugar and produce excessive gas (but, if you added a small amount of orange juice to the blend, this should not produce that effect).

Yogurt contains friendly bacteria and is easier to digest than milk by virtue of the fermentation process, which reduces the milk sugar component. However, yogurt is not recommended because of its high fat content, mucous-forming properties, allergenic proteins and its content of chemical and drug residues from commercially-fed cows.

The trouble with taking in an excess of bacteria from products and drinks is that they can overpopulate the alimentary canal and set up fermentation, especially when fruit is eaten. Bacteria in the gut eat stagnant fruit sugars, and this leads to fermentation and fatigue. If any such store-bought or homemade product causes bowel gas, the body does not need it and its use should be discontinued.

4.3
DEMYSTIFYING VITAMIN B$_{12}$

by Paul Fanny, H.D., Ph.D.
This article appeared in *Living Nutrition vol. no. 19.*

Understanding the Mechanics
of Vitamin B$_{12}$ Absorption

Vitamin B$_{12}$ (cobalamin) is a coenzyme which is produced by bacteria; it cannot be synthesized by plants or animals. The major function of vitamin B$_{12}$ is the promotion of growth and red blood cell formation.

There are several sources from which we can obtain vitamin B$_{12}$. It is available from some foods that go through the normal means of digestion with the help of intrinsic factor (a glycoprotein contained in gastric secretions), which facilitates the absorption of vitamin B$_{12}$ by the ileum mucosa.

Dr. Douglas N. Graham, author of The 80/10/10 Diet *book, states: "Since the beginning of time, humans have acquired some of their vitamin B$_{12}$ directly from fruits and vegetables. Since the advent of modern agriculture in 1942, when Bayer and other chemical manufacturers began diverting leftover chemical weapons from World War II into use as pesticides and fertilizers, farmers have inadvertently sterilized the bacteria out of our soils. The resulting loss of plant-derived dietary vitamin B$_{12}$ is just one of the unintended consequences. It is easy to understand why nutritional researchers generally encounter no vitamin B$_{12}$ in plant foods since they take their samples from produce grown in dead soils. However, organically grown plants specifically cultivated in highly composted soils rich with organic matter can contain plenty of B$_{12}$."*

According to Dr. William S. Peavy and Warren Peary's book, Super Nutrition Gardening, *there is evidence that adequate cobalt in the soil along with microorganisms provide the conditions for the production of vitamin B$_{12}$ in plants. Some land plant foods, including nuts, have been found to contain significant amounts of vitamin B$_{12}$. Under normal conditions, vitamin B$_{12}$ can also be manufactured and absorbed in the human absorbing colon as a result of bacterial activity. According to Gabriel Cousens, M.D., vitamin B$_{12}$ researchers Drs. Thrash and Thrash estimate that the microorganisms between the teeth and gums, around the tonsils, in the tissue at the base of the tongue, and the nasopharyngeal passages produce approximately 0.5 micrograms of vitamin B$_{12}$ per day. There must be adequate cobalt and other nutrients in the human body for the formation of vitamin B$_{12}$. These sources of bacteria (teeth, gums, tonsils, tongue and nasopharyngeal passages) that synthe-*

size vitamin B_{12} do not need intrinsic factor to carry vitamin B_{12} through the small intestine to the ileum. The vitamin B_{12} is absorbed through diffusion of their mucous membranes as is the case with vitamin B_{12} that is produced by bacterial activity in the colon and absorbed in the absorbing colon.

After vitamin B_{12} has been absorbed into the bloodstream, it is stored in large quantities in the liver and released slowly as needed to the bone marrow and other bodily tissues. According to Guyton and Hall's Textbook of Medical Physiology, *the minimum amount of vitamin B_{12} required each day for normal red blood cell maturation is only 1.0 to 3.0 micrograms, and the normal store in the liver and other body tissues is about 1000 times this amount.*

Again, according to Dr. Cousens, Harvard medical school researcher Louis Sullivan demonstrated that only 0.1 microgram of vitamin B_{12} is sufficient to evoke a physiological response from people who are vitamin B_{12} deficient. Most leading experts, says Dr. Cousens, conclude that 0.5 micrograms of vitamin B_{12} per day is sufficient for maintaining health. Dr. S. J. Baker, a laboratory researcher at Christian Medical College Hospital, reported that "the daily vitamin B_{12} intake from foods of vegetarian South Indian villagers resulted in vitamin B_{12} levels of 0.3 to 0.5 micrograms. They appeared to be healthy and did not show any signs of vitamin B_{12} deficiencies." According to Dr. Cousens' research, although vegans show a lower level of vitamin B_{12}, their absorption ratio of vitamin B_{12} (70%) is higher than that of meat eaters (26%) and, therefore, they do not need to absorb as much vitamin B_{12}.

As quoted by Dr. Cousens, Dr. S. J. Baker stated that "5.0 micrograms of vitamin B_{12} are produced in the colon per day and vegetarians receive more vitamin B_{12} from the reabsorption of bile than from foods eaten." Since humans need less than 0.5 micrograms of vitamin B_{12} each day, the content of vitamin B_{12} in bile secretion (1.0-10.0 micrograms) is a significant potential source (if it can be absorbed).

Why Adequate Gastric Secretions are Vital for Vitamin B_{12} Absorption

Why are adequate gastric secretions vital for vitamin B_{12} absorption? First, let us understand the physiology of gastric secretions. Gastric (stomach) secretions are produced by two types of tubular glands:

1. Oxyntic (acid-forming) glands, which are composed of parietal cells secreting hydrochloric acid, pepsinogen, intrinsic factor, and mucous, and

2. Pylori glands, which secrete mainly mucous for protection of the pyloric mucosa and pepsinogen along with the very important hormone gastrin.

It is crucial for the oxyntic glands to secrete adequate intrinsic factor which combines with vitamin B_{12} in the stomach. Intrinsic factor protects vitamin B_{12} from being destroyed by digestive enzymes while passing through the small intestines until it is absorbed by the ileum at the lower end of the small intestine. In the absence of intrinsic factor, it has been reported that approximately 1/50 of the vitamin B_{12} is *absorbed. Malabsorption of both vitamin B_{12} and folic acid may cause the lack of full development of red blood cells (maturation failure) and inevitably lead to anemia and other health-related problems.*

Causes of Inadequate Gastric Secretions Carrying "Intrinsic Factor"

Gastritis (inflammation of the stomach lining), in most cases, is the cause of inadequate gastric secretions and intrinsic factor, but this can also be symptomatic of disorders of the small intestine such as celiac disease, malignancies, drugs and many other related factors.

Causes and Developments of Gastritis and Its Results

Gastritis is frequently caused by a poor, nutrient-deficient diet of spicy, salty, and high-fat foods that are fried, boiled or baked, destroying vitamin B_{12} and mutating it to an inactive vitamin B_{12} analogue that cannot be absorbed by the cells. Other causes of gastritis may include: stress, liver disease, radiation poisoning, vascular injuries, direct traumas accompanied by lesions and some degree of hemorrhaging, severe burns, sepsis, shock, renal failure, infections associated with gastric ulcers, gastric adenoma carcinoma and renal disease. Additional causes, stated in Human Anatomy and Physiology, *which can destroy vitamin B_{12} produced by bacterial activity in the intestines, are high alkaline and acid conditions, such as those occasioned by drug use and the eating of animal flesh containing antibiotics.*

Chronic gastritis develops as the gastric mucosa slowly atrophies until little or no gastric gland activity remains. The loss of normal stomach acid secretions, specifically intrinsic factor needed for vitamin B_{12} absorption, leads to an impaired health condition called "achlorhydria" or "hypochlorhydria," wherein the stomach fails to secrete adequate hydrochloric acid and gastric secretions below a pH of 6.5. This usually leads to the development of pernicious anemia, which often accompanies achlorhydria, due to maturation failure of red blood cells in absence of vitamin B_{12} stimulation of the bone marrow.

Eliminating Vitamin B_{12} Deficiency: "Remove Cause, and There Are No Symptoms"®

We can greatly reduce the risk of vitamin B_{12} deficiency by discontinuing a toxic lifestyle of drugs, poisonous habits, stress, etc. These destroy the bacterial activity and other processes in the intestinal tract of the body.

Most researchers concur that the use of inactive vitamin B_{12} analogues ("fake" B_{12}, or "pseudo vitamin B_{12}") found in multivitamin supplements containing vitamin B_{12}, as well as spirulina, chlorella and blue green algae, can deplete, destroy and interfere with active (true) vitamin B_{12} by competing for the same cell receptor sites. (Analogues, as defined by Dorland's Medical Dictionary 27th Edition, *are chemical* *compounds with a structure similar to that of another but differing from it in respect to a certain component; it may have a similar or opposite metabolic action). In our quest for truth, it is important to differentiate between what is similar and what is authentic.*

Although some research has shown that blue-green algae contains ample, active vitamin B_{12} that is usable by the human body, the blue chromoprotein component which contains phycocyanin (an emetic), listed by James Duke in his Handbook of Biologically Active Phytochemicals and Their Activities, *is a protoplasmic poison and should not be ingested.*

Many types of seaweed (marine algae plants) such as nori contain inactive vitamin B_{12} analogues that are possibly harmful to people, especially if they are vitamin B_{12} deficient. Seaweeds that do contain active vitamin B_{12} would in most cases need to be eaten in the amount of 30 grams a day to secure enough active vitamin B_{12} through the digestive process. This is ten times the recommended serving and could cause other health problems due to the high intake of iodine and sodium chloride.

Testing Methods

Many researchers and scientists agree that there are many contradictions in the current testing methods and research between what is considered active vitamin B_{12} and inactive vitamin B_{12} analogues found in foods and humans. Dr. Stephen Walsh, a leading, modern-day vitamin B_{12} researcher, wrote an article on Algae and B_{12}, which can be found at http://www.scienzavegetariana.it/nutrizione/alga_ klamath_en.html under the subtitle "Characterization of vitamin B_{12} compound from unicellular coccolithophorid alga (Pleurochrysis carterae)." Dr. Walsh summarizes the research on the consumption of algae showing the evidence of acceptable levels of authentic vitamin B_{12}. He states: "The only acceptable test for a B_{12} source to be considered adequate is consistent prevention and correction of B_{12} deficiency in humans without impaired absorption." What he means to say is, even if there is an adequate source of active vitamin B_{12}, it doesn't matter if it can't be absorbed. Now allow us to restate Dr. Walsh's statement, adding emphasis to the key concept: "Only when absorption is unimpaired can we test for an adequate vitamin B_{12} source that is consistent with the prevention and correction of vitamin B_{12} deficiency in humans." This statement supports the Hygienic, Natural Health tenet: "Remove Cause (impaired absorption), and There Are No Symptoms."®

At an American Natural Hygiene Society Conference in 1979, researchers Dong and Scott took blood samples from 83 predominantly raw and cooked-food vegans who did not take vitamin B_{12} supplements. The incidence of macrocytic anemia (nutritional anemia) was found to be "minimal."

If, despite what you think constitutes a natural healthy lifestyle, you begin experiencing neurological problems, enlargement of the mucous membranes of the mouth, vagina and stomach or are experiencing macrocytic anemia, please consult *a Hygienic Health Professional. You could be vitamin B_{12}-deficient.*

The most reliable and natural testing method for vitamin B_{12} deficiency is the uMMA Test (urinary methylmalonic acid test).

Bodily Providence

The body is a self-healing, self-regulating marvel that works best when we do not interfere with its physiological and biological functions. This recalls the story of the intelligent body who one day grew tired of its Master meddling in its health affairs, loudly proclaiming: "Mind your own business, and I will mind mine."

Summary

Guyton and Hall's Textbook of Medical Physiology *states that "vitamin B_{12} deficiency is not normally due to a lack of vitamin B_{12} obtained from foods, but rather a malabsorption of vitamin B_{12} due to a deficiency of gastric secretions and intrinsic factor. It can also be a lack of folic acid." Dr. S. J. Baker stated: "Vegetarians need as little as 0.3 to 0.5 micrograms of vitamin B_{12} per day to avoid deficiencies."*

Various sources from which we can obtain vitamin B_{12} every day include: 1. foods containing vitamin B_{12} produced by bacteria on or in fruits and vegetables, providing sufficient vitamin B_{12} can be absorbed by the ileum mucosa through the normal means of digestion; 2. the bacteria producing vitamin B_{12} (0.5 micrograms) and its coenzymes in the mouth, teeth, nasopharynx, the tonsils and the tonsillar crypts, the folds at the base of the tongue and upper bronchial tubes, the throat, esophagus and the upper small intestines through the process of diffusion; and 3. in the colon, where bacterial activity produces approximately 5.0 micrograms of vitamin B_{12} per day, and which is absorbed by the absorbing colon through diffusion.

Under normal, healthy conditions, avoiding impaired digestion, diffusion and bacterial activity caused by drugs, poison habits and stress, active vitamin B_{12} will be manufactured and absorbed in the intestinal tract. Vitamin B_{12} deficiency will not normally occur in rawfood vegetarians and fruitarians who practice Hygienic, natural health living habits.

4·4
A GENERAL GUIDE TO FOOD SELECTION

by Dr. T. C. Fry

It is worth the health benefits to buy organically grown produce which is grown in living, naturally fertilized soils without the use of any chemicals. Commercially grown produce (non-organically grown) is generally grown in sterile, mineral-deficient soils, using chemical fertilizers, pesticides and fungicides, washed in chlorine solution (which kills most of the "friendly" bacteria), then treated with preservatives. Organic produce has been proven to contain higher quantities of vitamins and minerals, and generally tastes better than commercially grown.

One way in which to pinpoint the pathogenicity or salubriousness of foods is their metabolic endpoint character. Acid-forming foods are pathogenic unless offset with alkaline end-product foods. Most meals should consist of 100% alkalizing foods. One dinner salad meal a day with acidifying food should contain at least 80% alkalizing foods. Acidifying foods should never be eaten when there is internal inflammation or other illness. Foods that result in alkaline end-products are:

• *All raw vegetables.*

• *All raw fruits, including high-acid fruits such as lemons and oranges, etc., excepting blueberries, cranberries, plums and prunes.*

• *All fresh raw green beans, peas and their sprouts.*

Foods that result in acid end products are all heavy protein content foods including:

• *All meats including fish.*

• *All animal products including milk but excepting blood and butter. (We cannot get calcium from milk because it is tied up in the casein which later becomes soil for putrefactive bacteria.)*

• *All legumes or bean family members in their storage (mature, dried) form of proteins, fats and starches except fresh lima beans, fresh peas, green beans, soybeans and sprouted beans/legumes,. This includes peanuts, which are widely consumed. Lima beans contain a deadly poison, as do garbanzo beans.*

• *All nuts and seeds excepting almonds, chestnuts, fresh coconuts, pine nuts (pignolias) and sesame.*

• *All grains excepting amaranth, millet and quinoa.*

See Dr. Shelton's book Food Combining Made Easy *and our food combining chart.*

Criteria for the Selection of Best Foods

First Criterion - Can the food be eaten in its natural state? Is the food palatable, that is, delectable or delicious? Can it be eaten with keen relish in its natural state?

If a food cannot be eaten with joy and delight to individuals in normal health with unperverted tastes, then the food receives a very low rating or no rating value. Eating should be a gustatory delight. If a food is a taste delight, it receives a perfect score and a lower score commensurate with its delectability.

If the food cannot be ingested in its natural or raw state, that is, uncooked, unprocessed and otherwise untampered with, it does not belong in the human diet and receives a rating accordingly. We humans were for millions of years adapted to a diet obtained directly from nature in its fresh raw natural state. This determines the character of our diet and also the manner in which we were accustomed to ingesting it.

Therefore, cooking and processing foods to make them palatable is unacceptable to the Natural Hygienist. Cooking destroys enzymes totally. While a healthy individual will synthesize some 1,000 enzymes required for digestion, assimilation and utilization of foods, the body is, nevertheless, dependent upon the enzymic action of the foods for the most perfect digestion. Consequently, it is absolutely essential that our foods have their full complement of enzymes intact.

Cooking is the worst practice humans have adopted. It destroys not only the enzymes but deranges and destroys almost all known food factors. Cooking disorganizes, oxidizes and makes a food's mineral content unusable. It deaminizes the food's protein content thus rendering it worthless in human nutrition. Cooking reduces the value of a food from its wholesome state all the way down to worthless ashes, depending on the degree of cooking to which it has been subjected. To the extent that a food has been cooked—reduced to inorganic minerals, caramelized sugars and starches, coagulated and deaminized proteins, poisonous acrolein laden fats, devitalized vitamins and loss of fuel and other values—it is not only worthless but the ash becomes toxic debris in the body. That cooked foods are poisonous in the body is easily demonstrable. The white corpuscle count doubles and triples after eating them! So the rule is this: If we can't eat the food "raw," if it is not delicious and palatable in its natural living state, it is not a food for us!

RATING: 0 to 25 on our scale of evaluation.

Second Criterion - Does the food introduce harmful or toxic substances into our digestive system?

If the food is proper to the human diet, it must contain NO noxious or unwel-

come substances. We do not want poisons in our system, no matter how little or how "mild." Anything that interferes with vital activities or destroys cells and tissue is poisonous to our system.

RATING: 0 to minus (-) 100 on our scale of evaluation, depending on degree of toxicity.

Third Criterion - Is the food easy to digest and assimilate?

Foods to which we humans are ideally adapted require a minimum of vital energy necessary for their digestion and assimilation. To be of greatest value to us, foods must be efficiently digested and assimilated, granting, of course, that we have unimpaired digestive systems.

Humans have become highly efficient at digesting and assimilating foods to which they, in nature, became adapted. Millions of years of development made certain foods very easy to digest. We developed constitutions, enzymes and processes that appropriated, digested and assimilated certain foods with a minimum expenditure of vital resources and time.

RATING: 0 to 25 on our scale of evaluation.

Fourth Criterion - Does the food contribute a broad range of nutrients? Does the food possess great biological value for us?

I have appraised the foods listed herein for many factors. Though many foods are rather complete in their range of nutrients, none are suitable for a mono diet such as is for cattle. But most of the foods rated are quite suitable for mono meals. And, certainly, if properly combined, these foods furnish all the nutrients we humans need.

The problem is not that we should eat a great variety in hope of making sure to get all the nutrients needed, but, rather, to eat simply to afford our bodies every opportunity to easily digest and appropriate what the foods offer. What does it matter the range of nutrients we put into our bodies if we ingest them in such a manner as to vitiate and tax the digestive process so that, instead of appreciating our good intentions, we fail to derive the goodness intended and penalize our bodies and rob it of nutrients as well? We should never eat more than four or five different foods at a single properly prepared and combined meal. Almost no preparation other than cleansing is necessary, but we must make sure to eat in strictly compatible combinations. The ideal is a single food per meal! There is no particular penalty in eating two to four different items at a meal if they are compatible in the digestive process.

To really simplify the digestive process and to assure yourself of easy digestion on a continuing basis, we may select a rather narrow range of foods according to the season and stick with them. For instance, we may make one meal a day of just bananas with some lettuce and celery and another meal of a salad and nuts. This can go on day after day in the winter season. In summer we might have melon rather consistently for just one meal and at a second meal of the day, a salad with nuts or some fresh food of a starchy or proteinaceous character. The objective is a diet to which we are biologically adapted that gives the highest potential for wonderful health.

The ratings given herein are arrived at based on data available to me and my appraisal of it and other factors. I have taken into account the contribution to nutrition a food may make in the matter of calories, vitamins, minerals, enzymic factors, hormones, proteins, auxones and other beneficent food factors. Keep in mind that most foods are fairly complete in themselves if they are seeds or nuts, though this does not necessarily mean they are complete in human nutrition.

Green leaves must be accorded the highest and most complete range of nutrients. This is one of the primary reasons we must have them often in our diet for the best health (that is, if we're eating). Of course the body is provident—missing them on occasion is not particularly harmful and would not prove disastrous unless we missed them for some length of time.

While this rating chart does not spell out the nutrient contents—that knowledge not being necessary—we should plan our meals so that we receive the benefit of foods that complement each other in their nutrient contents essential in human nutrition.

RATING: 0 to 50 in our scale of evaluation.

Other Considerations Not Rated

Is the food acid-forming in metabolic reaction? Is it alkaline in metabolic reaction?

The value of a food in human nutrition is not determined by these considerations, but the human diet must consist overwhelmingly of alkaline-forming foods. Generally, nuts, legumes and cereals are acid-forming. Nuts are quite beneficial in the human diet, whereas humans do not have the equipment to properly digest legumes (except in sprouted or fresh green state) and cereals.

Is the food economical? Do we get good nutritive value for our money?

A food's value to us must also be gauged by its cost versus its utility. For instance, we can sprout mung beans and receive some of our best nutrition for just a fraction of the cost of the same values in other foods.

Is the food generally available in its fresh, natural state?

This, too, is a consideration. We must eat our foods as nature delivers them to us. We can make little use of foods that have been tampered with—ground, cut up, peeled, cooked, preserved, canned, frozen, etc. Even sun-dried foods are not nearly as wholesome as in their fresh state. Raisins, figs, dates, apricots and pears, for instance, are great foods in their fresh state with all their original water content. Dried, they lose much of their vitality but, on the other hand, they are not nearly as injurious as they would be if cooked. And they are excellent as fuel foods during the colder periods of the year. Their use in the warmer times of the year is unnecessary and ill-advised.

Summary of Rating Factors

1. *0 to 25. The food is rated according to its edibility and delectability in its fresh natural state.*

2. *0 to minus (-) 100. The food is rated for its harmfulness in the human diet. We should skirt as much as possible all foods that have within them unwelcome substances.*

3. *0 to 25. The food is rated according to its digestibility and assimilability.*

4. *0 to 50. The food is rated for its biological or nutritive value in human nutrition.*

Food Rating Chart

For best health, eat foods rated 80 or higher.

NAME OF FOOD	RATING CRITERIA				TOTAL
	(1)	*(2)*	*(3)*	*(4)*	
ALMOND	22	-10	22	47	81
APPLE	25	0	25	42	92
APRICOT	25	0	25	46	96
APRICOT (Dried)	20	0	20	40	80
AVOCADO	23	0	22	45	90
ASPARAGUS	15	-5	20	45	75
BANANA	25	0	25	48	98
BEAN (Green)	22	0	25	47	94
BEAN (Sprouted & Greened in Sun)	20	0	23	47	90
BEET	15	-5	15	42	67
BERRIES (Generally)	23	0	25	45	93
BRAZIL NUT	23	0	23	47	93
BROCCOLI	24	0	25	47	96
BRUSSELS SPROUT	22	0	24	46	92
CABBAGE	23	0	24	45	92
CANTALOUPE	25	0	25	47	97
CARROT	22	0	22	45	89

| NAME OF FOOD | RATING CRITERIA | | | | TOTAL |
	(1)	(2)	(3)	(4)	
CASHEW	10	-5	15	45	65
CAULIFLOWER	23	0	25	45	93
CELERY	25	0	25	44	94
CHERIMOYA	25	0	25	45	95
CHERRY (Sweet)	25	0	25	45	95
COCONUT	20	-5	15	47	77
COLLARD GREENS	22	0	24	48	94
CORN (Fresh Sweet)	25	0	25	45	95
CUCUMBER	20	0	20	40	80
CURRANT (Black)	25	0	25	46	96
DANDELION	15	-25	15	48	53
DATE (Sun-Dried)	25	0	25	40	90
FIG (Fresh)	25	0	25	48	98
(Dried)	25	0	25	42	92
FILBERT (Hazel Nut)	22	0	23	47	92
GRAPES (Generally)	25	0	25	47	97
GRAPEFRUIT	21	0	25	43	89
HONEYDEW MELON	25	0	25	47	97
KALE	23	0	23	48	94
LETTUCE, Romaine	25	0	25	45	95
Bibb	25	0	25	45	95
Iceberg	25	- 5	25	30	75
MANGO	25	0	25	47	97
MELONS (Generally)	25	0	25	41	97
OKRA	20	0	20	45	85
ORANGE	25	0	25	47	97
PAPAYA	25	0	25	47	97
PAW PAW	25	0	25	47	97
PEACH	25	0	25	46	96
PEA (Fresh Green Sweet)	25	0	25	46	96
PEANUT	12	-10	12	48	72
PEAR	25	0	25	45	95
PECAN	25	0	25	47	97
PEPITAS (Squash Seeds)	20	0	25	47	92
PEPPER (Sweet Red)	25	0	25	47	97
PINEAPPLE	25	0	25	47	97
PLUM	25	0	25	45	95
POTATO (Irish)	5	0	20	45	70

NAME OF FOOD	RATING CRITERIA				TOTAL
	(1)	(2)	(3)	(4)	
POTATO (Sweet)	15	0	20	45	80
RUTABAGA (Peeled)	20	0	22	42	84
SESAME SEEDS	15	0	20	47	82
SPROUTS (Alfalfa, Mung, Greened in Sun)	20	0	23	47	90
SQUASH	25	-5	25	45	95
SUNFLOWER SEEDS	20	0	23	47	90
TANGERINE	25	0	25	45	95
TOMATO	25	0	25	45	95
TURNIP (Peeled)	20	0	22	35	77
WALNUT	25	0	25	47	97
WATERMELON	25	0	25	45	95

4·5
KEY FOODS

Bananas: The Ideal Food For Humans

by Dr. T. C. Fry

Bananas deserve the highest rank as food for humans. It is one of the oldest foods of humans and has been treasured for its deliciousness. The ancients referred to the banana plant as the "Paradise Tree" and its fruit as the "fruit of paradise." Never has there been a more apropos description of a food. Bananas are one of our most important foods and deserve a far greater role in our diet—in fact, they should be our foremost item of diet as they are with many tropical peoples, who also eat other tropical fruits such as breadfruit, jakfruit, coconut, mango, etc. We are a class of frugivores that achieved our high development with fruits of the tree as the bulk of our diet. Fruits of the tree in our pristine habitat were mostly sweet fruits such as bananas, figs, grapes and dates.

In its general suitability and beneficence in the human diet, few foods approach the banana. It is, ecologically and biologically, our most ideal food. Dates, figs, grapes, melons and oranges, quite common foods, deserve a place in our diet, but in the final analysis, the banana wins on practically every count: economy, nutrition, convenience, plenitude, deliciousness, etc. Apples are a wholesome food, but they are woefully deficient in protein, having only 0.2% by dry weight and then only two or three of the essential amino acids, whereas bananas have all the essential amino acids and have about 5.2% protein dry weight.

Bananas are available all through the year. It is best to buy them organically grown and green for ripening at home, where ripening conditions can be controlled—you can try putting them in a brown paper bag overnight, and expose them to air during the day. Commercially grown bananas are usually picked long before they are ripe and nutritionally mature, and "gassed" with ethylene to facilitate ripening, as well as treated with such toxic chemicals as methyl bromide and aldicarb. Ethylene is the naturally occurring ripening gas produced by fruits; it is commercially synthesized by pyrolysis of hydrocarbons. Some organically grown bananas may also be gassed with ethylene, so your best chance for getting ungassed organic bananas may be to get them green. It also behooves you to ask your produce supplier if the bananas have been gassed, and to request ungassed organic bananas.

Select bananas free from surface bruises, with skin intact at both tips. Ripen at room temperature. When the skin is bright yellow speckled with brown, the starch has changed to fruit sugar, and the fruit will be tender sweet, and easy to digest. Fruit that ripens with brown speckles may not have been gassed, as I have been told that gassed bananas ripen with dark streaks and blotches instead of the brown speckles. I have found that speckled fruit is uniformly delightful in taste, so I am inclined to give some credence to this speculation.

I stress bananas as a major item in the diet primarily for reasons of overall goodness, availability and economy. It is of course beneficial to include other fruits as food, such as fresh figs, dates, grapes or some other highly nutritious fruits, plus greens, some sea soft vegetables and nuts.

Humans are frugivores to their very cores! We'll do best if we respect our natural disposition. The banana is one of the ideal foods in the human diet.

Greens

The term "greens" refers to a low-calorie, non-starchy, low-protein (on a per-bite basis) category of foods including: lettuces (green, brown and red) and other vegetable leaves such as bok choy, Brussels sprouts, cabbage, collards, kale, spinach and sunflower seed sprouts, plus broccoli leaves and crowns and celery stalks (or ribs).

In nature, all fruit-eating primates eat some greens. Greens are crucial to our health, providing an abundance of vitamins, minerals in electrolyte form and phytonutrients plus fatty acids, water, fiber and other nutrients. Greens function as the solar collectors of vegetables wherein phytonutrients are formed. The high mineral-to-sugar content of greens complements the sweetness of fruit and induces a balancing effect for those who are sensitive to sugar.

Greens are most nutritious in the fresh, young, tender raw state. When leafy greens are cooked, the majority of nutrients are damaged, deranged or totally destroyed. Light steaming (212 degrees F) certainly has a far less deleterious effect than does heating at higher baking temperatures. Tender greens, such as lettuce, should never be cooked. Greens in the whole form should not be eaten during the healing stage because of their high roughage content. It is best to juice leafy greens during the healing phase in combination with either sweet fruits or carrots and other vegetables.

After healing C&C, everyone's bowel muscle tone and digestive strength are relatively weak. As such, whole greens are typically not handled well or enjoyed during the first year by some people, except in spare quantities. However, as the body becomes stronger and healthier, more and more whole greens can typically be digested and enjoyed with good results. Thorough chewing is always an essential factor in digestion.

The greens which are suitable for sensitive digestive systems, during and after healing, when eaten in appropriate fashion as advised herein, include: tender, young, non-bitter lettuces and celery ribs.

Some greens have varying degrees of toxic, irritating components. None of the

following are appropriate during the healing phase:
- crucifers with high sulfur content: bok choy, broccoli, Brussels sprouts, cabbage, collards, kale, rutabaga and turnip
- leaves and stalks with high oxalic acid content: chard, parsley, purslane, rhubarb and spinach
- leaves with bitter components: arugula, celery (leaves), mustard, watercress and any others which taste or feel hot or sharp in the mouth

Several months after the healing phase, when all symptoms are gone and health is robust, the following mildly-irritating greens may be tested by gradually introducing them in moderation, if they are enjoyable: bok choy, broccoli, Brussels sprouts, cabbage, collards, kale, parsley, purslane and spinach. Always avoid the highly-irritating bitter and sharp greens: chard, rhubarb, arugula, celery leaves, mustard and watercress, plus leaves which are overly-mature, containing irritating alkaloids.

Dr. Herbert M. Shelton reported that greens are beneficial to the digestion of fatty, high-protein foods, such as avocados, nuts and seeds. As a predominate eater of fruit for 24 years, my daily diet regularly includes two heads of lettuce and two bunches of kale, substituting occasional bok choy, non-bitter salad mix and tender inner ribs of celery; I enjoy these immensely eaten whole and plain. A balanced sense of wellness is experienced when they are eaten with sweet fruits (except melon which is best eaten alone) and we are in a state of good health and fitness.

I also enjoy growing lettuces and kale in my garden. I simply sprinkle seeds in mineralized organic soil and add water. The young, tender leaves are most enjoyable when picked fresh. By allowing some of the plants to mature and go to seed, I am able to collect a bounty of seeds for next spring's planting.

In the "Ask the Nutritionists" column in vol. no. 20 of my *Living Nutrition* magazine, Dr. Douglas Graham wrote:

You do have to consume your greens—feel free to drink them. I have found that people who include insufficient greens in their diet invariably suffer health decline.

Greens provide a density of minerals that cannot be found in fruits. Of course, green leafy vegetables provide us with more than just minerals. They provide a wealth of essential fatty acids, fiber, pure water, protein, antioxidants and an exceptionally wide range of phytonutrients.

While it is not essential to eat greens every day, I recommend that 2% to 4% of total calories come from greens. If you only eat 1% or as much as 5%, you should still do well. It is healthful to blend your greens, but a good salad is a real joy. Be open to the possibility, for your likes and dislikes will change in time.

Young tender greens taste marvelous on their own. I love eating plain lettuce and celery, too. I sometimes eat several heads at one sitting.

In his book, *The 80/10/10 Diet,* Dr. Graham wrote:

Leafy greens and other vegetables, when eaten raw and fresh, contain a small amount of fatty acids in an easily-usable state. However, some (primarily cruciferous vegetables) contain unwanted toxic sulfur compounds. We derive our best predigested fats adequate to meet our fatty acid needs from fruits and tender leaves.

By every indication, our digestive physiology was designed to process the soft, water-soluble fibers in fruits and tender leaves, almost exclusively.

It is true that cruciferous vegetables like broccoli, cauliflower, kale, collards, Brussels sprouts and cabbages are loaded with nutrients, including soluble fiber. But they also contain cellulose and other difficult-to-digest or even indigestible fibers.

By "indigestible fibers," I mean that our digestive system cannot break down these materials and must therefore eliminate them. And unlike soluble fibers, these digestible fibers are rigid and may scratch and scrape our delicate digestive lining as they pass through. These vegetables are best digested when eaten in their youngest and most tender state. For best results, they must be thoroughly chewed or mechanically predigested via the use of a blender or shredding device.

To assimilate completely, we need to digest completely, and every time we eat foods that are difficult to digest, we compromise our nutrition and, over time, our health. Surely, we are capable of swallowing vegetation that contains cellulose and other rough, insoluble fibers, but such foods place a great load on our organs of digestion and elimination.

In vol. no. 18 of my *Living Nutrition* magazine, Dr. Graham wrote the following article:

Celery: More Than Worth Its Salt

Mention celery in any group of people and you will usually get very polarized responses. In general, most folks don't have very strong feelings about carrots, lettuce, cucumbers, or other vegetables, but when it comes to celery, it seems they either love it or they just plain hate it. And their reasons are as varied as are the characteristics of this many-splendored veggie.

Some cannot tolerate celery's stringiness. Just something about that texture makes them uncomfortable. Other people like it, referring to the strings as "Nature's floss." Crunchy and juicy, salty yet sweet, celery is an enigma in the vegetable kingdom. Celery's root is considered a delicacy, yet the leaves are toxic and bitter. Its "half-pipe" rib shape makes it perfect for dipping into spreads or filling with treats. Celery seems to go well with everything. People enjoy eating celery with nut or seed paté as much as they enjoy it with berries, dates, blended with bananas, in salad or as crudités. Celery boasts one of the lowest "calorie-to-bite" ratios of all foods, yet it is extremely satiating and nourishing.

Celery travels exceptionally well. It stays fresh through an extended range of temperatures, withstands pressure changes admirably and "lasts" quite nicely, even without refrigeration. Celery is more than just hardy, it's almost supernaturaL If the base of a celery "bunch" is put in water, not only will the celery stay fresh for weeks, it will actually resume growing.

But celery has a lot more than just good looks going for it. Nutritionally, it is a powerhouse, rich in alkaline minerals. It is refreshingly juicy, yet exceptionally low in calories. Among terrestrial plants, celery is considered one of the best sources of sodium. It is high in fiber, rich in phytonutrients, and contains antioxidants and vitamins galore.

Celery is exceptionally rehydrating, being high in both water and electrolytes. Thus, it is a wonderful food for those who are physically active. It supplies 18 different amino acids, including all 8 of the essential amino acids, making it an exceptional source of complete protein. Though the outermost ribs of celery can be tough and even woody, the inner ribs are exceptionally soft, tender and very easily chewed.

Celery is truly a food worthy of much praise. In a world where green foods are touted as some of the most nutritious on the planet, celery scores extremely high marks. Be sure to include this versatile vegetable in many of your soup, salad, and dressing recipes.

Avocado: The Fruit That Would Make Butter and Meat Obsolete

Avocado is more than just a tasty treat to be enjoyed in guacamole—it makes a hearty, satisfying meal when eaten alone, in salads and in other dishes. Most people who transition from a standard American diet to a vegan diet with avocado, nuts and seeds don't miss the animal foods because raw vegan plant fat is so satisfying as well as more nutritious than cooked fatty animal foods! In hundreds of thousands of cases, people who've adopted a vegan diet of predominantly raw foods with minimal or no cooked starches as part of a healthful lifestyle (including regular exercise and adequate sleep) have lost excess weight, overcome illness, gained new vitality and avoided the killer diseases which now plague our meat, bread, dairy, and junk-food-eating society. The fresh vitamins, active enzymes, organic minerals, soluble fiber, high water content and easily digested fats and proteins in avocados and other fruit and plant foods can help transform any sluggish, overweight meat eater into a slimmer and more dynamic person. Some of the leanest people I know eat the most avocados! Cooked foods such as bread, pasta, meat, dairy and junk foods are the villains that can keep an avocado eater from losing excess fat.

If your goal is to reduce your consumption or transition completely off meat and dairy, avocado may be the perfect way to satisfy your natural cravings for creamy nourishment. Dr. William Esser wrote in his *Dictionary of Natural Foods:*

The avocado is one of the most valuable foods which nature has given man. For those concerned about eliminating meat from their diet, this offers not merely a "substitute," but a food which is much superior in value for human maintenance. It is rich in protein and fat and comparatively higher than any other fruits in these elements. The fat is more digestible than animal fats.

Avocado is also known as the "alligator pear" because of the rough skin on some varieties. In the 17th and 18th centuries, the fruit was also commonly known as "butter pear." In tropical Central America, avocado trees have been growing wild for thousands of years, providing natives with a rich food. The Aztecs called the tree "Ahuacatl." Marauding Spanish armies changed this to "abocado" or "avocado," the now common English name.

According to *The Little Green Avocado Book,* there is strong evidence that avocado trees flourished 50 million years ago in what is now California, and avocados might have provided food for dinosaurs.

Today's avocados are derived from three natural races. The Mexican type (semitropical) produces small fruits, 6 to 10 ounces, having glossy purple, paper-thin skin when ripe. The Guatemalan type (subtropical) yields medium pear-shaped fruits which are first green, turning purple-black or coppery-purple when ripe, with a typically tough shell. The West Indian type (tropical) produces enormous, smooth, round, glossy green fruits of up to two pounds in weight. In the United States, 95% of the commercially grown avocados come from California, with small percentages coming from Florida, Louisiana, Texas and Hawaii. *The California Rare Fruit Growers Fruit Facts, Volume One,* reports that avocados grow well in valley and coastal California, as far north as Cape Mendocino and Red Bluff. Hybrid forms of all types are grown.

Avocado growing is relatively new in the United States. Avocados are available year-round. Harvest time depends on the variety. The Hass, the best known commercial variety, is a hybrid of the Mexican and the Guatemalan types and is picked from January into fall, depending on where it is grown.

The Little Green Avocado Book also reports that avocado trees are large evergreens of the laurel family, and there are about 400 commercial varieties of avocado. Some are: Bacon, Ettinger, Fuerte, Gwen, Hass, Nabal, Pinkerton, Reed and Zutano. Mexican types ripen in 6 to 8 months from bloom, Guatemalan types 12 to 18 months.

There are wide differences in the flavors of individual avocados, ranging from salty, to nutty, to sweet, with shades in between. If a fruit has been picked too early, it may be watery and unpalatable. If picked too late, some varieties develop a rancid flavor. If a Bacon avocado tastes like bacon, it is rancid. If an avocado has dark flesh (rot), compost it and/or salvage the good parts.

At some farmers markets and produce stores, one can occasionally find "Cukes" (also known as "Cocktail" or "Finger" avocados), seedless, pickle-shaped avocado fruits which result from improperly pollinated flowers. One can also occasionally find miniature avocados which have thin, black edible skin and an anise flavor (the Mexicola is one variety)—these make a delightful treat!

Julie Frink, Curator for the Avocado Variety Collection, University of California Research Station at Irvine, California, wrote:

I have nearly 20 varieties growing in my yard and the Hass variety is always one of the best. Some of the green varieties sold in stores have given a bad name to some really fine green-skinned fruits. The most inferior tasting avocados have either been picked when too immature or they are poor-quality pollinator varieties to begin with. One of our favorites is the round, green Reed. A perfect Reed on Labor Day is a most fantastic treat! So often these wonderful fall avocados are picked and sold in the spring when they are watery and tasteless. The green, elongated pear-shaped Pinkerton can be fantastic if allowed to stay on the tree until full maturity, but will be rubbery and tasteless if picked too soon.

The Little Green Avocado Book also states that an acre of avocado trees can yield more food than an acre of any other tree crop. Imagine the ecological implications—a perfectly healthful "meaty" food which requires 1/200th or less of the acreage needed by the cattle industry for a comparable yield in pounds, posing no pollution problems—and no carnage! Worried about mad cow disease?—eat raw avocados, seeds and nuts and stay sane and mentally keen!

Avocados are bursting with nutrients—vitamins, A, B-complex, C, E, H, K, and folic acid, plus the minerals magnesium, copper, iron, calcium, potassium and many other trace elements. Avocados provide all of the essential amino acids (those that must be provided by our diet), with 18 amino acids in all, plus 7 fatty acids, including omega 3 and 6. Avocados contain almost as much protein as mother's milk, about 5% caloriewise per edible portion. Since rapidly growing nursing infants obtain an average of 7% of their calories from protein from mother's milk, we can safely assume that children and adults do not regularly require foods richer in protein than avocado. Our bodies recycle approximately 80% of our protein; cooked protein is denatured and largely unusable, thus, our protein need is far lower than what is taught by conventional dietetics. A small avocado will provide more usable protein than a huge steak because cooked protein in meat is deranged and mostly unavailable to our liver, the organ which makes all of our body's protein. There is clear evidence from many sources that cooked fatty and high-protein foods are the prime culprit in our country's high rate of cancer, as well as in colitis, Crohn's disease and many other diseases. (I instantly healed from a long illness, ulcerative colitis, twenty-three years ago after I stopped eating meat and adopted a properly combined low-fat vegan diet of mostly raw fruits and vegetables, and I have since helped over 1,000 people recover from similar illnesses.) Ripe, raw organically grown avocados are naturally pure and furnish all of the elements we need to build the highest quality protein in our bodies.

The water content of avocado by weight averages 74%. Because avocado is a ripe, watery, enzymatically-alive fruit, it ranks as the most easily digested rich source of fats and proteins in whole food form. The ripening action of the sun "predigests" complex proteins into simple, easily digested amino acids. The fat content (by weight) varies from 7% to 26% according to the variety, averaging 15%. Approximately 63% of the fat in avocados is monounsaturated, 20% is polyunsaturated and 17% is saturated. Avocados are the perfect source of dietary fat—appetizing in their raw state, digestible and pure. Another plus is that avocados have no cholesterol.

Avocado is an alkalinizing food, i.e., the mineral end products of metabolism have an alkalinizing effect in the blood and other bodily fluids. Because the human body works to maintain a slightly alkaline pH, an alkalinizing diet is the most healthful way of eating. Meat, dairy and most raw nuts create acidity in the body—excess eating of these causes the leaching of alkalinizing calcium from our bones to buffer the acidity, leading to osteoporosis. Dr. Douglas Graham states:

Current bone density testing has verified loss of calcium from the bones after the consumption of just one meat meal. A similar meal containing the same amount of protein from plants results in no calcium loss. Fruit and vegetable proteins, which supply the complete spectrum of human nutrients, must be considered superior to animal protein, which is deficient or missing many of our essential nutrients such as fiber, vitamin C and a host of phytonutrients and antioxidants.

Avocado eaters who eat a healthful vegan diet typically experience more lustrous hair, softer, smoother skin, more pliable nails, fewer joint problems, slimmer belly, less body odor, improved mental function and enhanced libido. Upon giving up animal meat and dairy, switching to a diet of 75% to 100% raw vegan foods with enzymatically-alive "plant meat," and adopting a healthful lifestyle, a multitude of people have reaped amazing health benefits and joyous vitality.

How To Eat Avocado

Using your fingernails, peel off the skin. The skin of a naturally ripened avocado will easily spiral off in one to three pieces.

Alternatively, using a knife, slice an avocado along the north-south or east-west axis, then remove the pit. The halves can be sliced into smaller segments. The skin can then be peeled off, or you can scoop out the flesh with a spoon. Eat plain as a snack or scoop the flesh into a bowl or onto a salad.

Avocado generally requires approximately one-and-a-half to two hours in the stomach to be digested. It digests well if the eater is relaxed, hungry, energetic, has an empty stomach and follows proper food combining guidelines. If one eats avocado when tired, one may fall asleep.

For optimum digestion, eat avocado alone or with any non-sweet, non-starchy fruit or any non-starchy vegetable food. Eating avocado with leafy greens, celery and/or cucumber will enhance the digestive process as additional digestive enzymes are secreted. People with weak digestion will generally experience enhanced digestion when eating avocado with non-starchy salads as opposed to eating avocado alone.

Avoid eating avocado with or within 20 minutes of eating sweet fruit or drinking sweet fruit juice. The combination of a small amount of lemon or grapefruit juice with avocado tends to digest well for most people.

Wait at least 3 hours after eating avocado before eating sweet fruit.

Do not eat avocado with any other kind of oily, fatty or high-protein food such as seeds, nuts, coconut, olives, yogurt, cream, cheese or meat. Wait several hours between eating these foods, although the ideal time is 24 hours. It takes several hours to digest and utilize any kind of heavy/oily food, and the body can only digest one at a time.

Avoid eating avocado if you are experiencing bowel inflammation, acid reflux, indigestion, sore throat, pain or fever.

Overeating avocados can lead to sluggishness, hyperacid stomach, skin outbreaks and C&C.

The quantity of avocados that is healthful for you is a function of your taste preferences, digestion and health condition. Generally, one-quarter to one-half of a medium-size avocado a day, one to three days per week, is a good baseline for those who are in robust health. For those who have C&C or have recently recovered from C&C, begin with a spoonful with dinner one to three days per week and gradually increase the quantity if the results are positive. For best results, tune in to your body's senses and observe your energy levels, digestion and elimination.

Avocado Preparation Ideas
• Mash avocado ("avo butter") into baked potatoes
• Smear "avo butter" over steamed vegetables
• Dollop warmed "avo butter" over hot air popped corn
• Spread "avo butter" on whole grain bread and soft corn tortillas
• Dip baked corn chips into avocado halves, or a bowl of avocado pulp
• Halve and pit avocado then scoop (or "dip") celery, carrot, broccoli, bell pepper pieces in and eat as a snack
• Add spoonsful or slices to salads—there's your dressing!
• Mix with chopped bell pepper, tomato, celery, lemon juice, etc. for guacamole or salsa
• Party time: slice into spears or chunks, insert toothpicks and serve as hors d'oeuvres. (Who needs cholesterol and fat-laden cheese?)
• Make veggie "handwiches" or "veggie roll-ups"—place chopped veggies, sprouts, tomatoes and avocado chunks on lettuce, kale or cabbage leaves, fold them over or roll them up, and enjoy
• Add to processed vegetables—veggie slaw, veggie loaves, veggie cakes and cookies

• Mix into veggie and sprout soups—blend in to make a creamy texture, or serve "chunky style"
• Make dressings—avo-carrot juice, avo-tomato-celery (add a little lemon or grapefruit juice and/or herbs to taste)
• "Avo butter"—smear a halved avocado over freshly shucked corn on the cob
• Stuff avocado and veggies into cored bell peppers (whole or halved) and serve as a "handwich" or other entrée

Note: avocado and starchy foods (e.g., potatoes, bread, grains, corn, old carrots) make a "fair" food combination—for optimal digestion, do not combine avocado and starchy foods.

Avocado vs. Animal Meat

Avocado - Watery and fiber-rich, non-constipating
Animal Meat - Low water, no fiber, constipating

Avocado - Has all essential amino acids
Animal Meat - Amino acids denatured by cooking

Avocado - No cholesterol
Animal Meat - High in cholesterol

Avocado - Takes 2 to 4 hours to digest, normally will not putrefy
Animal Meat - Takes 12 to 24 hours to digest, normally putrefies, poisoning our blood, tissues and brain

Avocado - No parasites, pathogens or tumors
Animal Meat - Incidences of parasites, pathogens and tumors range from rare to common

Avocado - Not inoculated with any chemicals
Animal Meat - Typically inoculated with antibiotics, medicines and hormones

Avocado - Water-rich and non-allergenic
Animal Meat - Bloody and laden with allergenic proteins

Avocado - Does not need cooking nor any preparation other than peeling
Animal Meat - If eaten raw, the parasite-pathogen risk increases; when cooked, the fats become carcinogenic, the proteins coagulate, and the heat-deaminated minerals become embedded as arterial and bowel plaque leading to atherosclerosis, heart disease, Alzheimer's, etc.

Avocado - 100% healthful
Animal Meat - A major health hazard with links to cancer, colitis, diabetes, obesity and many other diseases

Avocado - Alkalizing
Animal Meat - Acidifying

Avocado - The fuel required to digest avocado and other fruity fats is less than half that required to digest meats, and digestion time is dramatically lower as well
Animal Meat - Takes approximately 50% of body's energy and as much as three days to digest and clean up the toxins from its decomposition in the gut and the immune system response to the toxic proteins and grease which enter the blood

Avocado - 100% ecologically sound
Animal Meat - Ecologically destructive, requiring up to 200 times the acreage and over 10 times the quantity of water to produce one pound of food (approximately 220 gallons of water per pound of avocado vs. 2,400 gallons water per pound of beef); grazing causes soil erosion and in some countries deforestation; liquid, solid and gaseous animal wastes pollute the atmosphere, land and waterways

Some Avocado Myths and Facts

Myth - It's a vegetable
Fact - It's actually an oily berry—a fruit

Myth - It's high in cholesterol
Fact - It has no cholesterol—only animal foods have cholesterol

Myth - It's high in fat
Fact - By weight, avocados average 30% easily digestible oily fatty acids and approximately 70% water

Myth - Its saturated fat content is dangerous
Fact - Only about 2.5% of the edible portion of avocado is saturated fat, and unheated saturated fat from live plant foods is nontoxic

Myth - It's fattening
Fact - It is the cooked starches, meat, dairy and processed sugar in people's diets that feed their fat cells. Most active people who consume avocados as part high raw food vegan diet have no problem losing excess fat and staying lean

Myth - It is a tree ripened fruit
Fact - The avocado doesn't soften on the tree. After dropping or picking, it must be allowed to soften for 4 to 17 days depending upon the variety and ambient temperature and humidity

Myth - It's best to ripen it in a bag
Fact - Not necessary. Keep your weekly supply of avocados on your kitchen table, counter or somewhere else in plain sight. Pinch the tops and bottoms each morning and when they yield to pressure on both ends they are ripe. Refrigerate the ones you are not ready to eat

Myth - It can't be refrigerated
Fact - Yes it can. Wrap ripe avocado in plastic or keep it in a plastic bag or container. If it is refrigerated for too long, some spoiling may result. Remove unripened avocado from the refrigerator 2 or 3 days before you intend to eat it

Myth - Keep the seed in to keep guacamole from turning black
Fact - That is an old wives' tale! Wrap it in plastic to keep oxidation at bay

Figure 2
Raw Food Pearamid
© David Klein, Ph.D.

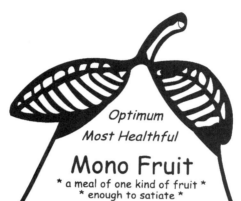

Optimum
Most Healthful

Mono Fruit
* a meal of one kind of fruit *
* enough to satiate *
* only on an empty stomach *

Multiple Fruits
* a properly combined meal *
* only on an empty stomach *

Fruit with Vegetables
* a properly combined meal *

Vegetables
* a properly combined meal *

Vegetables with Nuts or Seeds
* a properly combined meal *
*Least energising * Eat sparingly*

4.6
Understanding Hunger and Appetite

While preparing to write this section I sat down under a tree one day and made a list of reasons why people, including myself, eat. I stopped after I had identified 50 reasons, and over 40 were emotional in nature! Humans mostly eat out of emotional habit, equating their "appetite" with a strong message from their bodies that says: "Food! Feed me now and don't stop until I feel better!" Some people eat to satisfy this "appetite" believing they are filling a true need for nutrition, while others do so knowing that this is not the case.

You may believe you need to work on "controlling your appetite." When we recognize that we have an emotional eating problem, working on "controlling our appetite" rarely, if ever, works. The reason is we neither understand the nature of the "appetite" nor how to approach it. I do not believe that our "appetite" is something to control, but rather something to *understand.* Let's explore this and see how getting to the core of our reasons for eating can help us.

Understanding "Appetites"

"Appetites" can be considered to be desires which arise from thoughts, memories and bodily needs. The needs can be physiological (nutrients/food/water/sunshine/exercise/rest/sleep) or emotional (comfort/security/love). Emotional eating can and sometimes does help us to cope. However, food can never truly solve an emotional "appetite."

Essential and Non-essential Eating

There are only three essential reasons to eat: 1. to nourish our bodies when we experience true hunger; 2. to hydrate our bodies when we are thirsty; and 3. to fuel our bodies before and during rigorous work and exercise. Eating for any reason other than the three essentials is, to a greater or lesser degree, not healthful. How can we set ourselves free of unhealthful eating?

Body Awareness

The key to healthful eating is mindful body awareness. This practice leads to self-knowledge, which is the gateway to health, freedom and longevity. As conscious beings, we have the ability to develop our self-awareness on our pathway to self-mastery. With regard to eating, it is beneficial to observe our food cravings, appetites, food choices, the manner in which we eat, what our mind is doing while we eat, our emotions and our body's sensations during and after eating.

By practicing body awareness in a relaxed manner while we eat, we gain new insight about ourselves and our appetites. The magic of this is that as we come to know ourselves, we are constantly improving our ability to make healthful choices. Then, as our health blossoms, sickness becomes a thing of the past. We begin to feel great all the time, and we no longer stuff our stomach, intestines and colon, pollute our blood and brain, or waste our money on excess food. There is a tool for helping us become proficient at body awareness and getting to the core meanings of our "appetites." It is called...

The Somatic Inquiry

The Somatic Inquiry is a practice of sensing and observing the energetic presences and voids in and of the body, the inner terrain so to speak, and so discovering our true needs. In practicing the Somatic Inquiry you will naturally hone your ability to eat, live and care for yourself healthfully. By inquiring into your appetites, you will gain a deeper understanding of their nature, so that you can discern what is and is not true hunger. After a while it becomes easy and natural to integrate the Somatic Inquiry into your life–just like sensing the outside air temperature and deciding how much clothing to wear.

Guidelines

Sit in quietude and develop an internal "witness" who silently and non-judgmentally observes everything about yourself: your thoughts, emotions, sensations, circumstances, etc. In a relaxed manner, keep on observing and practicing being present in the body, every moment.

One or more times each day, while sitting in quietude, have the "witness" do a somatic inventory: from head to toe, or any direction, observe all of the qualities of the energies, sensations, feelings, emotions and voids you sense in your body. When you come to a strong or interesting presence, locate it in the body and delve or inquire into it via the Somatic Inquiry as follows: What is the temperature, shape, color, texture, density, space, movement of the energetic presence? Does it have a sound? Is there any message? If it is a void, can you delve into it? Stay with the energies or the void and delve deeper and deeper, without dwelling on or analyzing anything that comes up. A shift or resolution may occur as you sense-feel.

Keep practicing emotional-body awareness all day, even while talking to people at work or in any other situation. Sense the energies in your body and accept whatever is there, observe how it wants to move and shift, and allow it all. Sometimes there will be a message in what we are feeling, and it'll be safe to express it to ourselves or others. When circumstances rule this out, we can always use our breath, exhaling deeply, allowing the emotional energy to flow through us, releasing it to the universe. Breathing is a great tool!

Practice the Somatic Inquiry when you have food cravings/appetites. Focus on the energies in and of the body. This helps us become comfortable with and accept the emotional body. This practice is about developing self knowledge—getting in touch with our true needs and appetites. Inquire into the nature of your "hunger appetite"—become aware of all of its sensations and feelings. Is it located in your stomach area? What do you feel? Tune in and observe the feelings and qualities—sense the energetic presence as a whole.

If you are having a "hunger appetite" in your belly, is your stomach region giving you a clear food signal? Maybe it is uncomfortable and just flexing. If you stay with it, the craving may shift and resolve to something else. If you drink a glass of water, that flexing might go away and you will have learned that the flexing was not actually hunger. Maybe your stomach is empty and just wants love—eating is not the answer; food is not love, but caring for your emotional needs is loving. How can you distinguish a need for love from a need for food? Invite feelings of love in and see what happens.

If you sense something uncomfortable in the belly, or experience low energy and a "blue" mood, this can trigger a sense of weakness, low self-esteem or neediness, leading to the habitual emotional response of eating sweets to boost your blood sugar, or fatty foods to fill up the sense of emptiness. Inquire into these feelings, too. The healthful goal is to eat only to satisfy true hunger. What does that feel like? In general, true hunger is a sensation we feel in the back of the throat when we have not eaten for a while; it is not a stomach sensation. Explore the sensations that arise when your stomach is empty and find your true hunger. Here is how to proceed:

Do you have a feeling somewhere that is calling for a specific type of food? Locate it in your body and get to intimately know it. Does your body want something creamy, or tangy sweet, or semi-sweet, or salty, or crunchy, or chewy, or juicy, or a combination of those? Do you recognize the food it wants? If you do, and if it is available, observe the food—sniff it, peel it or break it open if necessary. Sniff in the aroma some more. If the food is totally appealing, deeply feel the pleasant sensations in your body, then slowly and consciously bite and chew it. As you eat, observe the sensations and how you feel as the food goes down. Relax into the eating and digestion process, stay tuned in and keep on observing how you feel. Continue to eat until you are satiated, following your body's signals that your stomach is sufficiently (not completely!) full. Your appetite may shift, or the taste may change. It's best not to eat past those "stop signals." Put the remaining food in the refrigerator, compost it, or share it with a friend.

If you have difficulty with the process of getting in touch with your inner signals, this may indicate that you need to detox further, work with a coach, or just keep practicing on your own. Living on juices or water fasting helps clarify our windows of perception; emotional contractions/armoring and dense-body dullness will open up to heightened sensation and perception. Juicing and fasting also helps us overcome appetites for cooked food.

After you have finished eating, observe for several hours how you feel. Notice your energy, any pleasant and unpleasant feelings in your body, any indigestion. Do you feel happy, balanced, unbalanced, energized, sleepy, moody? Are you experiencing an appetite or craving? If so, locate it in the body and inquire into it.

The Use of Self-knowledge

File away all of this information in your memory and refer to it the next time you sense an appetite or craving. As you continue sensing and observing your body and evaluating all of your experiences, you will optimize your progress on the healthful eating path!

I wish you expanding enjoyment in your explorations of the inner terrain. The Somatic Inquiry is the most empowering and transformational dietary tool I know of; it can be more enjoyable than any artificial entertainment or outer-world adventure because it is real, it is alive, and it takes you to new fascinating dimensions of the wonderful you!

4.7
Vegan Healing Diet Guidelines

Notes:

1. During the healing phase (when C&C symptoms are present), complete rest at home or at a Natural Hygiene health care facility is recommended—healing occurs only when we rest and sleep. People with active flare-ups who are working, caring for family members or are in school are advised to arrange to take a sabbatical and get complete rest until health is restored. If after reading the following section you are unsure about how to proceed, consult the author or another hygienically-trained health coach or doctor.

2. As previously explained, weight loss will ensue as you clean out and nourish your body with this most healthful diet. The weight that is lost is actually toxic morbid matter, which has been making you sick, as well as unhealthy fat and water, so it is a good thing that your body has the wisdom to get rid of the debris that has been dragging you down! If you understand the healing process and the purpose of detoxification and are relaxed as you follow this program, your weight will bottom out at a level which is safe, at which time you will be clean inside; then healthy weight will gradually be regained, leaving you feeling genuinely healthy, happy, strong and free of disease. Indeed, it is not fun being very thin, but that is typically what we have to endure for a while as the body accomplishes its rebuilding task. Keep in mind that healing and rebuilding require patience; on this program you will be building superior health and there is no shortcut to health. If you need support during this phase, again, the author will be happy to assist.

3. If you are extremely thin, emaciated, anorexic and/or anemic when beginning the healing diet, consult your medical doctor, the author and/or a hygienic physician for guidance. The high-calorie fruits (whole, blended and/or juiced bananas, papayas, grapes, sweet apples, etc.), as well as mineral-rich fresh vegetable juices and steamed vegetables, sweet potatoes and squash, eaten whole or as soups and broths, are most beneficial for those conditions, supplying the fuel and nutrients needed by the body to regenerate and rejuvenate.

• Implement the Vegan Healing Diet as soon as is comfortable. An immediate change to a vegan diet is the quickest way to proceed with self-healing C&C. Fruits and vegetables will taste more and more naturally delicious as you become clean inside. If you need to make a gradual transition to a vegan diet, that is fine—begin by eliminating red meats, pork and fried meats. As soon as possible, discontinue all animal products (all animal flesh including poultry, fish, eggs and dairy), heated/fried oils, grain/flour products (bread, rice, pasta, oatmeal, etc.), chemical additives and preservatives, salt (including sea salt), spices, white sugar, coffees, caffeinated teas, pasteurized drinks, soft drinks, sports drinks, irradiated foods, non-organic and non-whole foods and supplements, fermented products, nuts, seeds, caramelized and crystallized dried sweet fruits, junk foods, chlorinated and fluoridated water, alcohol and recreational drugs.

• Temporarily (until your bowels are healed and you feel well) stop eating all vegan fatty high-protein foods: nuts, seeds, avocado, durian, olives, coconut and soy. Fatty foods prevent healing and perpetuate inflammation. Protein does not heal you, and there are adequate amounts of protein in most fruits and vegetables. Everyone can heal well on the Vegan Healing Diet, so there is no need to be concerned about protein.

• Temporarily discontinue eating raw vegetables, except in fresh-made juiced form—raw fiber (roughage) is antagonistic when C&C is present.

• Discontinue all supplements. Supplements are stimulating, usually not absorbed, and not what the body is designed to function well on. Exception: if you are being treated for a critically low nutrient deficiency, follow your doctor's advice.

• The individual's needs and taste preferences dictate the transition rate and food choices. Diabetics need to avoid fruit juices and eat whole fruits or fruit blended with celery or lettuce. Those with severe flare-ups, diarrhea and spasms may feel discomfort with all-fruit meals at the outset of the diet transition as the body cleans out; if this occurs, focus on whole fruits, primarily ripe bananas, get extra sleep and minimize juices until the offending old toxic matter in your bowel has passed and you feel better.

• Follow your advising medical doctor's advice with regard to medication; however, inform him about your healing diet plans and ask him or her to support you in tapering off the medications at a safe rate. Immunosuppressants are of no use in any case—they suppress healing and should be discontinued as soon as is safely possible.

• Do not rush into an all-juice or all-fruit diet—for some people this brings on too rapid detoxification. However, if you have a fever and your gut is in turmoil and cannot hold down any solid food, a temporary diet of fresh-made juices and smoothies is generally beneficial. Do not eat any heavy foods, such as nuts and seeds. Get the right healing guidance. The author will be glad to help.

• Just before and during eating, it is necessary to be calm and not preoccupied. Food should be eaten slowly, there should be plenty of fresh air and breathing should be free and not shallow. If possible, it can be beneficial to do some type of light exercise, such as walking, 15 minutes before eating in order to stimulate the body's metabolism. Similarly, 15 or 30 minutes after eating, a relaxing walk may also help oxygenate the blood and enhance digestion.

• Persons with advanced C&C may have trouble tolerating meals which contain different types of food. For them it may be beneficial to go for a period eating mono meals, i.e., meals with only one type of food (e.g. puréed banana, or melon). Symptoms of indigestion may subside in this way. Then more foods can be slowly added to the diet.

• Eat sweet fruit in the morning, mid-day and mid-afternoon if desired— whole and/or juiced and/or blended into smoothies. Consume enough to satisfy. Sweet fruit choices include: ripe bananas (the skins must be spotted—this is the best food for C&C), papaya, grapes (avoid tart varieties), soft (ripe) pears, melon, peeled apples, cherimoya, plums, raisins and dates (soaked if they are very dry). Avoid citrus fruits, pineapples, peaches, nectarines, berries (except blueberries), tomatoes and tomatillos—these acidic fruits generally cause too rapid detoxification and are irritating while there is internal inflammation.

• Avoid raw vegetables (except juiced) and tough skins of fruits. Peel your apples (except when juicing them). Eat pears when they are soft (ripe); their skins may be eaten or sliced away.

• Keep your body well hydrated with purified water and fresh juices. At least 1/2 gallon of fluids is recommended each day.

• Begin experimenting with fresh-made fruit and vegetable juices—one or two glasses per day, taken in the mid-afternoon or later. To avoid gastric distress, do not eat sweet fruit or drink sweet fruit juices or smoothies soon or later in the day after drinking vegetable juices.

• Eat solid food only if you are hungry. Learn to follow your taste buds and other senses and select and eat those vegan foods that taste delicious—those are the foods that will be most nourishing for you. Sniff your food before eating. If the sensation is pleasurable, you are ready to eat; if you do not receive a pleasurable sensation, that food will generally not be nourishing for you at that time—try other foods or inquire as to whether you are truly hungry. Learn how to tune into your body's hunger signals. While eating, if the experience or food becomes unappealing or you feel satisfied, stop eating; do not overeat.

• Raw foods are most healthful when eaten correctly; steam cooking is least destructive to nutrients. Heating food above about 118 degrees F destroys the food's life force, enzymes and most vitamins. High baking temperatures cause minerals to pop out of the plant cells, rendering them unusable and detrimental as they can become bound up in arterial plaque and cause edema. While raw juices, salads, or blended salads may be more nutritious, eating lightly steamed vegetables, soups and broths can be a most beneficial way to get mineral-rich vegetables into the diet. Avoid roasting, microwaving, sautéing and stir-frying (fried oils are most destructive to our health). Baking temperatures are higher than steaming temperatures and, thus, more destructive to nutrients. During the healing phase, avoid baking and use a steamer to cook if you desire cooked foods. Steam vegetables, sweet potatoes and squash just to the point where a fork can be poked through in order not to totally destroy the fiber and nutrients. During the healing phase, the most healthful cooked foods are steamed vegetables (celery and carrots), squashes and sweet potatoes.

• Cooked grains are unnecessary and not recommended—they are mucous-forming (setting up fermentation which causes flatulence, fatigue and brain fog), acid-forming (except for amaranth, millet and quinoa), clogging, constipating, sedating and require hours for digestion as the body attempts to convert the starches into sugar. For more information, read *Grain Damage* by Dr. Douglas Graham (sold by Living Nutrition).

• Avoid hot, spicy and irritating foodstuffs such as curries, spices, black pepper, cayenne pepper, onions, radishes, mustard greens, garlic and chili peppers—these will exacerbate existing conditions and can trigger flare-ups.

• Follow food combining guidelines to a "t." Eat fruit only on an empty stomach. Eat melons alone. Eat citrus fruits before sweet fruits. Do not eat fatty/protein foods (seeds and nuts, including coconut) with sweet fruit or starchy foods (squash, potatoes, carrots and corn). Legumes are poorly digested and not recommended; sprouted legumes are somewhat more digestible, yet are of marginal value and not recommended during the healing phase. Starchy foods combine well with all vegetables and non-sweet fruits except tomatoes—do not mix tomatoes with starchy foods. High protein/fatty foods combine well with non-starchy vegetables and cucumbers. Avocado combines well with any kind of vegetable, tuber and non-sweet fruit. Eat avocado minimally or not at all until you have completely healed. Review the Food Combining Chart on page 4-81 often until you know the rules by memory.

• Do not drink more than a few sips of juices or water when eating solid food. It is best to drink water or juices 20 minutes before eating solid food, and to wait one to two hours after eating solid food before drinking again (so as not to dilute your digestive enzymes).

• Chew your food slowly and thoroughly, 30 to 60 chews, mixing in your salivary enzyme secretions to assure optimal fiber breakdown, release of nutrients and digestion. This will ease the digestive work required by the stomach and other digestive organs. If solid food particles reach the small intestine, they can scrape the delicate membranes and decompose, causing distress.

• As the digestion of food and its transit through the stomach and bowel occur in a sequential manner, it is beneficial to space out meals at a minimum of three to five hours. Conversely, frequent meals can impose a constant drain of energy. Spacing out meals will allow time for the body's energies to focus on other tasks such as healing. Juicy fruits digest within minutes, while the denser fruits such as bananas and dates require about 60 to 90 minutes in the stomach. Starches require 4 to 6 hours. Fatty high-protein foods require about 6 to 12 hours. If the gut is in distress and bowel movements are occurring frequently, it will be impossible for the starches and fatty high-protein foods to digest completely—they will decompose in the gut, causing more gastrointestinal distress while impeding healing.

• Cultivate self-awareness about your eating and plan out your food choices. Eat consciously and only when relaxed. Do not eat solid food when tired or emotionally upset.

• Do not eat within two hours of bedtime. Do not eat a large meal within three hours of bedtime.

• Organically or biodynamically grown foods are the most nutritious and safest foods—eat the best foods you can obtain. Shop at healthfood stores and farmers' markets if available, buying the freshest fruits and vegetables.

• Make a gradual transition to 75% raw-living foods, or higher, for optimal health.

• Eat to support your body's efforts to create excellent health. Eat for bodily purity, mental clarity, perfect digestion, consistent, balanced energy and high vitality.

• If you are going to a place where healthful food will not be available, bring your own.

• Observe your stools—they tell you how well you have digested the foods you have chosen.

• Do not place any healing faith in food. Food has no healing power. Your body-mind has all of the healing power and does all of the magnificent healing work.

• Choose to live and eat healthfully, following your natural instincts. Each day affirm that your dietary transition is an unfolding process that will improve your life in wonderful ways and give yourself the patience and nurturing love you deserve.

• Study these guidelines every day until you know them perfectly.

Figure 3
Food Combining Chart

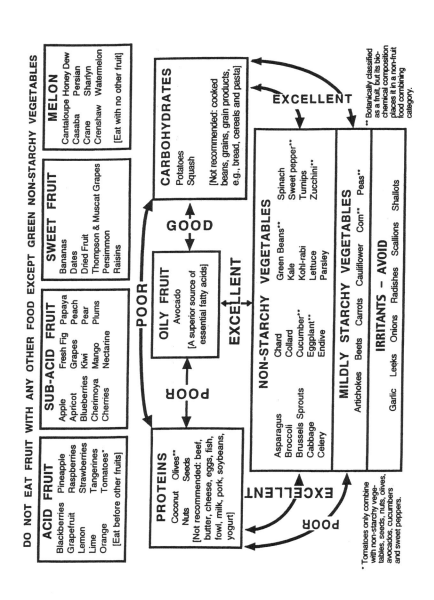

4.8
HEALING DIET MORNING AND DAYTIME MEAL CHOICES

Below are food choices for the morning, midday and afternoon as well as dinner, if desired. Always drink one to two glasses of water 30 or more minutes before breakfast. It is best to eat simply, consuming one (but no more than three) of these foods or items per meal. Always choose the sweetest, most delicious, ripe fruits. Bulky fruits can be eaten whole, mashed, puréed or blended with water or juice. Avoid acidic fruits, cooked foods and whole vegetables. Eat and drink enough to satisfy. Keep well-hydrated, include celery juice as often as possible and keep your energy level up by eating every two to three hours as is comfortable.

Always eat melon on an empty stomach with no other foods. Remove and do not eat tough skins. Apple skins may be juiced. Eat only ripe fruits. Bananas are the best healing phase food choice—the skins must be spotted. Variety is not necessary during the healing phase—go with what you enjoy and what works best.

If juices and juicy fruits increase diarrhea and discomfort to an intolerable level, avoid them until your stools become more solid and consume the denser fruits in whole or blended form, that is: banana, papaya, mango and soaked dates. If all foods and drinks cause distress, eat minimal portions of banana and papaya or whatever fruits work best and get complete bed rest. If you are struggling and unsure of how to proceed, contact the author.

Fruits

- Banana
- Papaya
- Melon
- Grape
- Cherimoya
- Custard apple
- Sugar apple
- Rolinea
- Breadfruit
- Plantain
- Lychee
- Rambutan
- Eggfruit
- Mango

- Apple
- Pear
- Apricot
- Loquat
- Sapote
- Persimmon
- Mamey (Mamea)
- Sapodilla
- Pawpaw
- Jakfruit
- Cucumber (peeled and de-seeded)
- Date (soak if very dry)
- Raisins (soak if very dry)
- Fig (soak if very dry and cut off the fibrous skin parts)

Fresh-made Juices

- Apple or apple-celery
- Grape or grape-celery
- Pear or pear-celery
- Apple-pear-celery
- Apple-pear or apple-pear-celery
- Melon

Fresh-made Fruit Smoothies/Blends/Soups

Any fruit listed above blended with your choice of water, celery juice, fresh coconut water, fresh-made juice, soaked dates or soaked raisins. Strain as needed to remove solids. The most highly recommended choices are:

- Banana-water (or banana-coconut water)
- Banana-celery juice
- Banana-date-celery juice
- Papaya-water (or papaya-coconut water)
- Papaya-celery juice

4.9
HEALING DIET
DINNER CHOICES

If you prefer and/or can only handle more sweet fruit for your last meal of the day, that is OK—the following choices are not essential; they may be introduced later:

Fresh-made Vegetable Juices

Drink fresh vegetable juice in the afternoon at least two hours after your last sweet fruit meal and no sooner than one-half hour before a dinner of steamed vegetables, potatoes and squash. Here are the choices:

• Carrot
• Carrot with choice of celery, cucumber, lettuce, red/yellow bell pepper
• Celery
• Celery with choice of cucumber, lettuce, sweet red/yellow bell pepper

Steamed Vegetables, Sweet Potatoes and Squash

Prepare the foods to be steamed by slicing them into bite-size slices or chunks. After steaming, the foods may be eaten whole or further prepared in any of the following ways, as desired:

• mashed with a fork
• puréed
• blended/puréed with water or celery juice, reheated if desired and eaten as soup
• blended/puréed with water or celery juice then strained, reheated if desired and eaten as a broth

Here are the food choices—they may be eaten alone or in any combination:

• Carrot
• Celery
• Squash (all)
• Sweet potato
• Yam

4.10
JUICE HEALING DIET

Notes:

1. An all-sweet-juice diet is not recommended for diabetics. For diabetics, sweet fruits must be eaten whole or blended with celery juice and/or lettuce.

2. Do not begin an all-juice diet until you have become comfortable for at least one week on the Vegan Healing Diet. Because rushing too quickly from a fatty, cooked-food diet to an all-juice diet often causes drastic detoxification, this must be avoided.

After you have become comfortable with your transition to the vegan diet, and your symptoms have diminished and stabilized somewhat but are still lingering and not reducing further, you can try an all-juice diet for one to five days, depending on how you feel. A diet of 75% juices and 25% sweet juicy fruits is also beneficial, in lieu of all juices. The all-juice diet is also prudent for those who are unable to hold down any solid food. You must take complete rest during this time.

This juicy diet will give your bowel a rest and enable it to heal up more rapidly. Most cases of lingering bleeding are healed via an all-juice diet for a few days. If you are interested in a water fast of more than 24 hours, see Appendix C and/or contact the author for a referral to a professional Hygienic fasting doctor.

To break the all-juice diet, begin with juice in the morning then one or two meals of solid or blended fruits later in the day. Continue this for another day or two, increasing the portion of solid fruit in your diet as is comfortable. If any bleeding has stopped, you can reintroduce steamed vegetables, potatoes and squash on the third or fourth day after breaking the all-juice diet. If lingering symptoms are not healing, you may simply need more rest and time on the all-juice diet. Obtain blood tests including mineral profiles to determine if there are any deficiencies. Most mineral and protein deficiencies are easily resolved without supplementation via the Vegan Diet—refer to section 4.2 for information on the richest food sources of specific nutrients, and increase your intake of them. Contact the author if you need guidance.

Refer to the previous two sections for juice choices.

4.11
POST-HEALING VEGAN DIET GUIDELINES

Begin the Post-healing Vegan Diet program approximately one week after all C&C symptoms (including blood and mucous) have ceased, stools are formed, evacuation is comfortable and regular (one to three bowel movements per day) and you feel well. Here are basic guidelines:

• Study and follow this healthful diet plan for a lifetime of health. It will always apply because your body has already demonstrated that unhealthful eating causes poor health including C&C. The price for falling back, that is, reverting to your old diet with cooked fatty foods, will likely be an even more severe/acute C&C crisis. This can occur at any time—even many years later—after healing C&C.

• Avoid expanding your diet too quickly. Your body will give you feedback about your limitations as you try new foods and larger quantities. Expand your diet gradually and avoid adding toxifying foods and overeating even the most healthful foods.

• Your gut will be extra sensitive for several months and it must be treated with extra special care. The colon needs a gentle workload as it rejuvenates. Bear in mind that the portions of your gut which were inflamed and, in some cases, ulcerated, have new tender flesh and, possibly, scabs which require rest for regeneration to take place. This means eating a high water content diet of mostly juicy fruits and tender vegetables, as opposed to a diet of excessive low-water content foods with a lot of roughage.

• Eating too much bulk/roughage/fibrous foods (such as raw vegetables, hard nuts, seeds and comfort food snacks, such as popcorn and rice cakes) will enervate the bowel and undermine the healing that has taken place. Bleeding and/or a flare-up can be triggered as the passing bulky mass scrapes the tender spots or scabs in the bowel. Large fecal masses can also stagnate at weak spots (strictures, bends or kinks) in the bowel, causing extreme discomfort, constipation, irritation, inflammation and a flare-up. If you ever get into such a situation, the healing protocol is to get onto a "cleaning out" diet of water, juices and juicy fruits and get extra rest and sleep until your bowel is healed. Our dietary errors are learning experiences—now you know what to do to heal and keep healthy!

• Eat to maintain unnoticeable digestion, clean bowels, minimal flatulence and peak energy.

• A diet of 75% to 100% raw foods with 75% to 90% fruit, including the non-sweet fruits (cucumbers, bell peppers, tomatoes, squash and avocados), promotes optimum health.

• Eat lightly in the morning—juicy fruits are energizing and most healthful—and the denser fruits after the first or second meal.

• Focus on eating the foods your senses find to be most visually attractive, fragrant, flavorful, refreshing and satisfying.

• After you are healed, you may gradually introduce sweet, ripe citrus fruits, such as oranges and tangerines, as well as ripe, sweet pineapple. These are best eaten at breakfast. The low-sweet and high-acid citrus fruits are generally too harsh when eaten during the first year after recovery from C&C—that is, your gut may be tender after years of inflammation and may not tolerate the acidic juices of fruits well for a while. After a year or more of healthful living, you will likely tolerate grapefruit and other acidic fruits. Lemons and limes are extremely acidic, harmful to tooth enamel, and best juiced and blended with fresh-made salad dressing if desired.

• If you are an athlete, body builder or engaged in rigorous physical work, take it easy for the first six or more months—exercise at a greatly-reduced pace so as not to stress your body, exhausting its energies while it is trying to accomplish the critical task of regenerating itself and establishing a new high level of health. Conserving your energy during the first 6 to 12 months will pay great dividends!

• If you are eating cooked food, do so only at dinner and always have a bigger portion of raw vegetables with it. For optimal energy and internal cleanliness, eat no more than one cooked meal per day and make that your dinner.

• Work on eating only when you are truly hungry, that is, when your body is sending a signal that it needs fuel. Become aware of emotional and other habitual eating patterns.

• Practice mindfulness as you prepare and chew your food.

• Chew your food thoroughly, mixing in your salivary juices until liquefied. Use a food processor if you are unable to chew well.

• Remember that simple is best, and work on resolving any overeating tendencies.

• If you experience constipation, that indicates that your digestive system and bowel need a rest. As such, sleep and rest more, drink more water, consume a simple, high-water-content diet of juices, smoothies and/or solid juicy fruits and avoid bulky salads, fatty foods and cooked foods until your bowel has regained vigorous energy. Fatty foods (avocado, nuts and seeds) and large bulky meals tend to be the main dietary causes of constipation.

• If sweet fruit is appealing but makes you feel unbalanced, minimize the sweet fruit portions while eating it with cucumbers, celery and/or greens. It may also be helpful to take a short water fast to improve your digestion.

• Follow these six keys to eating sweet fruit meals:

1. Exercise beforehand. Eating fruit (or any food) when we have no cellular need for the sugar and other nutrients can lead to metabolic problems.

We need to create the need for nutrients (true hunger) by exercising.

2. Clean out with water beforehand (10 minutes or more before eating). A clean alimentary canal will promote optimal digestion; a soiled alimentary canal leads to fermentation of fruit sugars, mucous production, indigestion, and food drunkenness or fatigue.

3. Eat sweet fruits alone (mono or combo) or combine them only with greens, celery and/or cucumbers (except melons—eat them alone). Sweet fruits digest and need to assimilate quickly. Sweet fruits (except melons) digest well with only the "neutral" green foods (i.e., foods which are low in protein or starch and, therefore, do not require a long time for digestion in the stomach).

4. After eating nuts, seeds, starchy vegetables or cooked food, wait until the next morning to have sweet fruit again. Those heavy foods require hours of digestion in the stomach and an hour of time is needed for them to pass through the intestines. There is one sweet fruit exception: acidic fruits can be eaten with and after meals with fatty foods (but not after any meals with starchy foods).

5. Eat sweet fruits with greens, celery and/or cucumbers to mitigate overeating on sweet fruits (if you have such a tendency). Rather than filling up on the sweet fruits, eat a small portion of them, then some of the green foods—alternate handfuls or eat together as desired.

6. Eat melon, especially watermelon, slowly and in small quantities if large quantities cause stomach discomfort or fatigue.

• People who have had C&C generally do not digest fats well. Therefore, high-protein, fatty and oily foods must be minimized, especially during the first year of recovery. Learning to eat within your digestive limitations is paramount. Fat intake must be increased gradually only in accordance with what you can properly digest. Overeating on nuts, seeds and avocados will, typically, stress the digestive system and create a toxic condition indicated by gas, foul, putrid bowel odors, stomach acidity, constipation, fatigue, etc., which can trigger a C&C flare-up.

• One or perhaps two ounces of nut or seed blends or butters eaten with one dinner salad meal per day may be all the fat that anyone can digest effectively after healing C&C. Similarly, two to four ounces of avocado may be one's digestive limit.

• Raw (ungerminated) nuts are difficult to digest; however, when eaten in small quantities (one ounce per meal, once per day, one to three times per week, depending on your digestive strength) and chewed well with lettuce, celery or cucumbers, they might digest well and give healthful benefits. The masticating action of our teeth is not capable of effectively breaking down hard nuts and seeds to particle sizes small enough to be completely digested by our stomach acids. Stomach acid can only act on the outer surface of particles; if acidic digestive enzymes are not able to act on the protein within the particles, the protein will pass through the system unused and will putrefy in the bowel.

• Raw nut and seed blends (made with water, citrus fruit or vegetables in a blender) and raw nut and seed butters (made in special juicers and available in jars from healthfood stores and by mail order) are much easier to digest than unprocessed whole nuts and seeds, and are, therefore, recommended. Still, they are very rich in oily fat which can cause problems if eaten beyond your digestive capability.

• "Living" nuts and seeds, i.e., raw nuts such as almonds germinated in water for 12 to 24 hours then sprouted in room temperature air, are more digestible than ungerminated (raw) nuts. The soaking and germination process hydrates and softens the hard fiber and reduces complex proteins into readily digestible amino acids. Germinated nut and seed blends (or patés) are perhaps easiest on the digestive system—simply blend one to two ounces of nuts or seeds with water, fresh-squeezed orange juice, a slice of orange or a tomato in a blender, then use this as a salad dressing or dip for vegetables.

• Experiment making nut and seed milks. Soak raw nuts or seeds in purified water for 2 to 24 hours, rinse well, blend at high speed with purified water in a blender, then strain and slowly drink the milk, mixing in your saliva.

• Avoid old rancid nuts and seeds—these tend to feel soft, taste cheesy with no sweetness and appear darker in color than when fresh.

• Heated or roasted nuts and seeds are very toxic and must be avoided. Avoid roasted and salted nut and seed butters.

• Peanut butter is not recommended because: 1. in raw or heated form, it is difficult to digest due to its high protein and starch content; 2. in roasted form it is highly toxic; and 3. peanuts are one of the most heavily pesticide-sprayed crops.

• Organic, whole, raw peanuts can be eaten in moderation if they have been sprouted (soaked in water and allowed to germinate for several hours). However, these are subject to a toxic, yellow mold and must be carefully inspected and eaten with caution.

• Olives are not recommended if they were cured in salt to remove the bitter alkaloids because too much salt remains in the olives. Some merchants offer raw olives which were cured via sun drying—these may be eaten if they are enjoyable. (Drying substantially changes the flavor, imparting an earthy character.)

• Hard, mature coconut pulp and flakes are not recommended because of the high starch and saturated fat content. The fresh, immature, gelatinous pulp from Thai ("green" or "young") coconuts is a healthful alternative.

• Bottled oils are not recommended—they are essentially one nutrient: liquid fat. Bereft of fiber, water and other nutrients, straight oil is highly congesting, that is, it thickens our blood and lymph and wreaks metabolic havoc. For optimum health, we must obtain our oils (fatty acids) from whole foods.

• Do not eat fatty meals (those including nuts, seeds, coconut or avocado) more often than four times per week. During your first six months of rejuvenation, you may do best on only one or two fatty meals per week. Even after you have gained robust health and good digestion, you may still do best on only one to two fatty meals per week. (The author thrives on one small fatty meal per week and experiences fatigue and various symptoms when he eats fat more frequently and/or in higher quantities.)

• To enhance digestion, eat fatty foods with cucumbers, celery and/or greens.

• If you sense that you need more satiation and energy from food to get you through the day and sustain you to dinnertime, eat larger meals and/or drink smoothies with the high-calorie fruits: bananas, papayas, dates and raisins. This helps quash the desire to overeat on fatty food at dinner.

• Avoid harsh irritating spices (e.g., pepper, cayenne, oregano, curry), condiments such as vinegar and pungent foods and herbs: pepper, oregano, onions, radishes, radish sprouts, garlic, arugula, etc., as these will irritate the most tender, most vulnerable parts of your gut, causing irritation and escalating to C&C. As a rule of thumb, if a food or additive burns your mouth, it is not fit for consumption.

• Minimize or avoid vegetables and roots which contain oxalic acid (which is irritating to the gut): parsley, chard, spinach (some spinaches are low-acid and may be OK in the diet on an occasional basis), rhubarb, purslane and beets. Oxalic acid also binds the calcium in those foods, making the calcium unavailable.

• Avoid all salt, including sea salt—inorganic crystalline salts are toxic and irritating to our tissues and cause many disease conditions. Salt cravings will disappear as you detoxify and nourish your body with fresh vegetable juices and vegetables.

• Avoid junk food treats. Fried and salted corn chips and fried banana chips are two examples of snack food you will find at health food stores which may appear to he healthful, but fried and salted foods are major health robbers. Make healthful treats from whole raw vegan foods—refer to the raw food recipe books offered by Living Nutrition and other sources.

• Avoid fermented foods. They contain toxic irritants, cause mucous and gas production and the strongly-seasoned ones lead to disordered eating.

• To assist in remineralizing your body, good sources of minerals are organic vegetable juices, vegetable salads, rinsed sea vegetables and barley grass powders.

• Observe your stools—they tell you how well you have digested the foods you have chosen.

• The Vegan Diet is the most healthful way to eat and thrive. If you are not getting the excellent results you desire, it is prudent to get coaching from a Hygienic counselor, such as the author. Countless people have succeeded and, with the right help, you can, too! Choose to be healthy for life!

4.12
POST-HEALING DIET
MORNING AND DAYTIME MEAL CHOICES

Approximately one week after all C&C symptoms (including blood and mucous) have ceased, stools are formed, evacuation is comfortable and regular (one to three bowel movements per day) and you feel well, you can begin the Post-healing Vegan Diet. During this phase, you can continue with all the Vegan Healing Phase Diet foods (included again below for convenience and marked with one dot) and carefully introduce the post-healing foods, which are listed below and marked with two dots. Avoid frozen fruit dishes if they cause discomfort.

Fruits

- Banana
- Papaya
- Melon
- Grape
- Cherimoya
- Custard apple
- Sugar apple
- Rolinea
- Breadfruit
- Plantain
- Lychee
- Rambutan
- Eggfruit
- Mango
- Apple
- Pear
- Loquat
- Apricot
- Sapote
- Persimmon
- Mamey (Mamea)
- Sapodilla
- Pawpaw
- Jakfruit
- Cucumber (peeled and de-seeded)

- Date (soak if very dry)
- Raisin (soak if very dry)
- Fig (soak if very dry and cut off fibrous skin)
•• Peach
•• Nectarine
•• Cherry
•• Cactus pear
•• Kiwi
•• Guava (Fejoa)
•• Tomato
•• Citrus fruits (orange, tangerine, mandarin, grapefruit, lemon juice, lime juice)
•• Pineapple
•• Pomegranate
•• Durian
•• Frozen sweet fruit "ice creams": banana; banana-fig; banana-date; papaya; mango; cherimoya; persimmon; jakfruit; durian; apricot; melon; etc. Optional: add a sprinkle of raw carob powder or topping of fruit sauce, raisins or chopped dates.
•• Frozen acid fruit sherbets: peach-plum; berry-cherry; cherry-tart apple; nectarine-peach; pineapple-tangerine, etc. Optional: top with berries.

Fruit Plates

Top these with a compatible fruit sauce or a sprinkle of raw carob powder if desired.

•• Sliced banana, grape and date on a bed of lettuce with diced celery and/or sliced cucumber
•• Sliced banana and papaya with fig sauce on a bed of lettuce with diced celery and/or sliced cucumber
•• Sliced banana and blueberry on a bed of lettuce with diced celery and/or sliced cucumber
•• Sliced apple, apricot and pear on a bed of lettuce with diced celery and/or sliced cucumber
•• Melon cubes or balls
•• Orange and tangerine segments and kiwi slices with diced celery
•• Pineapple chunks and tangerine segments on a bed of lettuce with diced celery
•• Berry, sliced peach and nectarine on a bed of lettuce
•• Tomato and cucumber with lettuce, kale or bok choy
•• Tomato and red bell pepper with celery, lettuce, kale or bok choy

Fruit Blends/Soups/Sauces/Dressings

•• Banana with choice of soaked date, fig, raisin, raw carob powder and lettuce
•• Mango with carob powder and celery
•• Mango, red/yellow bell peppers, lemon or lime juice
•• Mango with carob powder
•• Soaked fig, apple, celery
•• Soaked fig, red grapes, lettuce
•• Soaked date, pears, lettuce
•• Apricot, date, celery
•• Persimmon, date, celery
•• Pineapple and orange
•• Cherry and tart grape
•• Strawberry and mango
•• Tomato, cucumber and red/yellow bell pepper with lemon or lime juice
•• Tomato, celery and kale

Fresh-made Juices

• Apple or apple-celery
• Grape or grape-celery
• Pear or pear-celery
• Apple-pear-celery
• Apple-pear or apple-pear-celery
• Melon
•• Orange
•• Orange-pomegranate
•• Orange-tangerine
•• Grapefruit
•• Grapefruit-orange
•• Pineapple-tangerine
•• Pineapple-coconut water
•• Peach-plum
•• Cherry-tart apple
•• Nectarine-peach

Fresh-made Fruit Smoothies/Blends/Soups

These can be made from any single fruit or compatible fruit combination listed above, blended with a compatible choice of water, celery juice, fresh coconut water, fresh-made juice, soaked dates, soaked raisins, raw carob powder, celery,

lettuce and kale. Here are some choices:
- Banana-water (or banana-coconut water)
- Banana-water-raw carob powder
- Banana-celery juice
- Banana-date-celery juice
- Papaya-water (or banana-coconut water)
- Papaya-celery juice
- •• Banana-date-persimmon
- •• Banana-strawberry-water
- •• Pear-apple-celery juice
- •• Grape-banana-celery juice
- •• Apple-grape-celery juice
- •• Mango-water
- •• Mango-coconut water
- •• Mango-water-raw carob powder
- •• Mango-red bell pepper-lime juice
- •• Cherimoya-water
- •• Fig-banana-celery juice
- •• Fig-coconut water
- •• Apricot-banana
- •• Persimmon-dates-water
- •• Persimmon-water-raw carob powder
- •• Guava-tangerine juice
- •• Orange-Thai coconut pulp-raw carob powder
- •• Pineapple-strawberry-coconut water
- •• Blueberry-peach
- •• Raspberry-plum-fennel
- •• Blackberry-plum-mint leaf
- •• Tomato-celery-avocado
- •• Tomato-cucumber-kale-lemon
- •• Tomato-spinach-avocado-lemon juice
- •• Tomato-cucumber-collard greens-fennel

4.13
POST-HEALING DIET DINNER CHOICES

More sweet fruit may be eaten for dinner if desired. Or you can compose your dinner from the following raw and cooked food choices, eaten in proper combinations:

Raw Salad Ingredient Choices

These can be prepared in any appropriate ways: sliced, shopped, diced, minced, shredded, grated, julienned, spiralized, processed into noodles or thin spaghetti, etc.

- Celery
- Cucumber
- Lettuce
- Sweet red/yellow bell pepper
- •• Artichoke heart
- •• Asparagus
- •• Basil
- •• Beet
- •• Bok choi
- •• Broccoli
- •• Brussels sprout
- •• Cabbage
- •• Carrot
- •• Cauliflower
- •• Celery root
- •• Cilantro
- •• Collard greens
- •• Corn
- •• Dill
- •• Fennel
- •• Gooseberry (ground cherry or poha)
- •• Green bean
- •• Jerusalem artichoke (sunchoke)
- •• Jicama
- •• Kale
- •• Mint
- •• Okra
- •• Parsley
- •• Pea
- •• Rutabaga

•• Sea vegetables, rinsed
•• Snow pea pod
•• Spinach
•• Sprouts: bean and seed
•• Squash (any)
•• Taro root
•• Tat soi
•• Tomatillo
•• Tomato
•• Turnip

Steamed Vegetable, Potato and Squash Choices

Prepare the foods to be steamed by slicing them into bite-size slices or chunks. After steaming, the foods may be eaten whole or further prepared in any of the following ways, as desired:

• mashed with a fork
• puréed
• blended/puréed with water or celery juice, reheated if desired and eaten as soup
• blended/puréed with water or celery juice then strained, reheated if desired and eaten as a broth

• Carrot
• Celery
• Squash (all)
• Sweet potato
• Yam
•• Artichoke heart
•• Asparagus
•• Beet
•• Bell pepper, red/yellow
•• Broccoli
•• Brussels sprout
•• Cabbage
•• Cauliflower
•• Celery root
•• Collard greens
•• Corn
•• Green bean
•• Jerusalem artichoke (sunchoke)
•• Kale
•• Okra

•• Pea
•• Rutabaga
•• Snow pea pod
•• Taro root
•• Turnip
•• White potato

Baked Choices

It is best to minimize the quantity of baked foods in the diet—steaming is a less deleterious form of cooking.

•• White potato
•• Sweet potato
•• Yam
•• Squash (all)

Whole Grain Choices

It is best to avoid grains. If you choose to include any, it is prudent to minimize the quantity. Except for corn, all of these can be sprouted, rather than cooked. Grains can be cooked in a pot with vegetables, potatoes and squashes.

•• Amaranth
•• Barley
•• Corn
•• Millet
•• Oat
•• Quinoa
•• Rice
•• Rye
•• Sorghum
•• Spelt
•• Triticale
•• Whole wheat berries

Fresh-made Vegetable Juices

• Carrot
• Celery
•• Carrot with choice of celery, cucumber, red/yellow bell pepper, greens, beet and cabbage
•• Celery with choice of cucumber, red/yellow bell pepper, greens, beet and cabbage
•• Tomato with choice of cucumber, celery and greens and lemon or lime juice if desired

Nut and Seed Milks

You can experiment in your kitchen making nut and seed milks from raw and germinated sunflower, pumpkin and sesame seeds as well as almonds, pecans, macadamias, pistachios, etc. The milks are nutrient-rich, bountiful in easy to digest proteins and fatty acids, and mild-tasting yet delicious, without the mucous formation that results from ingesting cooked/pasteurized milk products.

Make sure the nuts and seeds you obtain are not rancid (soft, yellowed and cheesy-tasting) or heated (ask the supplier about the drying temperature—118 degrees F is the maximum for enzyme and nutrient preservation). Presoaking for at least two hours (12 hours maximum to prevent oxygen starvation) improves digestibility and releases bitter toxins from the skins of almonds and pecans.

Rinse, then blend with water and/or any of the following items at high speed until milky-fine: orange or pineapple juice, tomato, red or yellow bell pepper, greens. Use a nut milk bag to strain. Alternatively, use a fine-mesh strainer, pushing the liquid through with a large wooden spoon. Pour more water on top to release more milk, then push again. These milks actually make a complete meal. Avoid combining with sweet additives. Sip slowly and enjoy!

Wait 30 or more minutes if having a salad. Avoid starchy and sugary foods for several hours after ingesting nut milks to assure optimum digestion. Whole sweet citrus fruits, however, generally can be eaten 30 or more minutes after these milks with good results—their acids help break down fat and protein in the milks (these will mix in the upper sections of the gut).

Fatty Salad Ingredients

Use these in moderation and in proper combinations. Prepare them as dressings or add them to salads in whole or sliced form.

•• Avocado
•• Nuts
•• Seeds
•• Thai coconut pulp
•• Sun-dried olives (unsalted)

Salad Dressings, Sauces, Dips, Spreads or Side Dishes

•• almond butter-orange juice
•• almond butter-kale-cucumber-lemon juice
•• almond-pineapple juice
•• avocado-cucumber-grapefruit juice
•• avocado-carrot juice

•• avocado-tomato-basil
•• avocado-tangerine-fennel bulb
•• avocado-fresh corn niblets-zucchini-lemon juice
•• avocado-celery-kale-lemon juice
•• avocado-tomato-spinach-water
•• Brazil nut-grapefruit juice
•• flax seed-grapefruit juice
•• hazelnut-basil-grapefruit juice
•• hemp seed-orange juice
•• macadamia nut-orange juice
•• mango-red bell pepper-lime juice
•• pecan-grapefruit juice
•• pecan-guava-grapefruit juice
•• pecan-red/yellow bell pepper-orange juice
•• pine nut-grapefruit juice-basil
•• pine nut-tomato-basil-lemon juice
•• pistachio-lemon juice-water
•• pistachio-tomato-water
•• pistachio-tomatillo-parsley-water
•• pumpkin seed-grapefruit juice-celery
•• pumpkin seed-tomato-celery-lemon juice
•• sesame tahini-raspberry-orange juice
•• squash kernel-tomato-celery
•• sunflower seed-tomato-lemon juice
•• sunflower seed-basil-lemon juice
•• sunflower seed-dill-lemon juice
•• sunflower seed-tomato-dulse
•• sunflower seed-sunflower seed sprout-lemon juice
•• sunflower seed-pineapple juice
•• Thai coconut pulp-orange juice
•• walnut-celery-red/yellow bell pepper
•• walnut-celery-grapefruit juice
•• walnut-gooseberry-celery-water

Dinner Choices

Remember: 1. if you generally prefer sweet fruits and greens for dinner, that is perfectly OK; 2. minimize the meals with fatty and starchy ingredients to one to four times per week, in quantities that you can digest; 3. you can minimize the quantity or completely omit the fatty and starchy ingredients from any of the recipes; 4. always eat a raw salad with cooked foods; 5. simple is always better than fancy and complex; 6. properly combine the ingredients (e.g., do not mix nuts, seeds, sweet or acid fruits with starchy foods); 7. chew well; 8. do not overeat. For more recipe ideas, see the following section and order *Raw 'n Delish Vibrant Recipes* and our other recipe guides.

•• Greens salad, with mango-red bell pepper-lime dressing.

•• Tomato, red/yellow bell pepper, cucumber, celery and lettuce salad, served plain.

•• Garden salad with avocado, nut or seed dressing.

•• Greens salad with red/yellow bell pepper, with avocado, nut or seed dressing.

•• Your choice of celery ribs, carrot sticks, cucumber slices, broccoli crowns and/or broccoli florets scooped into a halved avocado.

•• Celery ribs and cucumber slices filled or topped with nut or seed butter or "cheese," served with a garden salad with tomato.

•• Tomato, greens, sprouts and avocado salad.

•• Tomato, greens and squash salad with avocado dressing.

•• Tomato and greens salad with nut or seed butter dressing.

•• Tomato, tomatillo and greens salad topped with soaked sunflower seeds.

•• Grated or processed raw vegetables, topped with avocado slices or served as a slaw with avocado dressing.

•• Veggie "handwiches":

    •• Slices or chunks of avocado, tomato, etc. rolled in large lettuce, kale or cabbage leaves.

    •• Almond butter spread onto large lettuce leaves, topped with tomato and shredded vegetables and sprouts, then folded.

    •• A halved red/yellow bell pepper stuffed with tomato, shredded lettuce and avocado, or nut or seed butter or "cheese."

•• Nut or seed milk, followed one-half hour or more later by a non-starchy garden salad with tomato-grapefruit juice dressing.

•• Thai coconut pulp blended with the coconut water, followed one-half hour or more later by a non-starchy garden salad with tomato-orange juice dressing.

•• A raw gazpacho of processed vegetables, sprouts, tomato and lemon juice, topped with whole or sliced cherry tomatoes and chunks of avocado.

•• A raw "pizza" (or "lasagna") with a thin "crust" of soaked then ground almonds, topped with a paste of raw and soaked, dehydrated tomatoes with basil, then topped with a freshly-processed pine nut "cheese," served with a garden salad.

•• Raw or steamed sweet corn smeared with avocado, followed by a salad of greens and red/yellow bell peppers.

•• Fresh-made zucchini and beet "spaghetti," served with a garden salad with avocado dressing and a baked potato with "avocado butter."

•• Steamed vegetables, potatoes and squash, served with a garden salad with avocado dressing.

•• Steamed vegetables and baked potato with "avocado butter," served with a garden salad with avocado dressing.

•• Steamed broccoli with nut dressing, served with a non-starchy vegetable soup and a non-starchy salad with seed dressing.

•• Steamed cauliflower with avocado dressing, served with a salad with avocado dressing.

•• Steamed sweet potato or yam, served with a cold or hot vegetable soup and a garden salad with avocado dressing.

•• Baked spaghetti squash, served with a garden salad with avocado dressing.

•• Frozen peas thawed in hot water, served with a garden salad with avocado dressing.

•• Frozen corn niblets thawed in hot water and served with a garden salad with avocado dressing.

•• A medley of pot-cooked vegetables, squashes, potatoes and one grain, served with a garden salad with avocado dressing.

4.14
SELECT FRESH RECIPES

The following recipes were taken from 300 recipes in the *Raw 'n Delish Vibrant Recipes* book edited by the author. They are generally fancier than the ones provided in the previous sections; however, they are provided to show you the simple gourmet possibilities of raw food eating. Not all of these recipes are for everyday use and some may be too rich and complex for your consumption in regular portions—if so, minimize the quantities or simply pass them by. Nevertheless, all of them can help entice your family and friends in the direction of healthful raw food eating. Experiment, improvise, obey your body's digestive limits and enjoy what you can!

Nut Milk

Almond Milk *by Phyllis Avery*
Serves 2

3/4 cup of raw almonds, soaked overnight and rinsed
2 cups of cold purified water
optional: raw carob powder

Finely grind the almonds in a blender. Add 1 cup of water to the blender, blending for 1 min. Slowly add the remaining water, blending for 1 more min. Optional: add carob powder to taste. Strain the mixture and serve.

Sweet Treats

Fruit Rolls with Mango Lime Sauce *by Christina Chadney*
Serves 2 for side dish, or 1 for a meal.

Sauce
1 mango
1/2 lime

Filling
1 mango, julienned
1 med. cucumber, seeded and julienned
1/2 med. or 1 sm. avocado, julienned
a few sprigs of fresh mint, finely minced
a few sprigs of fresh whole leaf cilantro

Wrap
1-2 heads baby bok choy leaves, rinsed and stems removed

Place a bok choy leaf face down on a cutting board. Layer strips of fruit—avocado, mango, cucumber—in center of leaf. Sprinkle with cilantro and mint, then roll tightly, using a toothpick to fasten. Arrange on a plate with a small bowl of dipping sauce. Variations: Papaya is a nice addition to the filling. Romaine lettuce leaves make a nice wrap if bok choy is not available.

Fudge Pudding or Ice Cream *by Dr. Douglas Graham*
Blend equal parts date and banana in a food processor. Add water sparingly if needed. Spoon into bowls and enjoy. To make ice cream, add frozen banana to the food processor with the dates, or add room-temperature bananas then freeze after processing. Note: A large quantity of dates will keep the mixture from freezing solid. Optional: Add raw carob powder and vanilla to taste. Add other chopped or small pieces of dried fruit for an interesting texture and added flavor

Berry Good Pie *by Dr. Douglas Graham*
Crust
approx. 2 pints of ripe strawberries

Filling
approx. 1 pint of blueberries
approx. 1 pint of blackberries

Topping
pulp from 1 Thai coconut
pulp from 1/2 very ripe pineapple
2 handfuls of raspberries

Blend the strawberries and pour into a pie dish, spreading evenly. Place layers of blueberries and blackberries on the crust. Blend the coconut pulp and pineapple together and pour it over the berries. Decorate with a ring of raspberries. Freeze and serve.

Salads

T. C.'s Super Salad *by T. C. Fry*
Serves 4 to 6

2 to 3 lbs. of tomatoes
4 avocados (or 1 lb. chopped or ground nuts or seeds)
4 stalks of celery
4 lg. red or yellow bell peppers
2 lbs. bok choy greens
optional: 1 grapefruit

Dice the tomatoes, celery and bell peppers. Quarter, peel and dice the avocados. Cut up the bok choy. Place all ingredients in a bowl and mix together. Optional: squeeze the juice from the grapefruit over the salad.

Raw Straw Slaw *by Dr. Douglas Graham*
Serves 2

6-10 ribs of celery, shredded
1 avocado
1 orange, juiced
handful of strawberries

Mix or blend the celery with the avocado and orange juice, then top with strawberries.

Winterfest Salad *by Living Nutrition*

peeled and sliced kiwifruit
segmented satsuma, mandarin, Fairchild and/or honey tangerines
segmented blood oranges
diced celery

Mix all ingredients in a bowl and serve on a bed of lettuce.

Perfect Low-Fat Salad *by Living Nutrition*
Serves 2

2 heads Boston (bibb) or butterleaf lettuce and/or other greens
1 lg. red bell pepper, chopped
juice from 1/2 lime (ripe limes are light yellow-green, not dark green)

flesh from 2 lg. or 4 sm. mangos
juice from one blood orange or other orange
optional: 1 fennel bulb, chopped

Place the greens in a large bowl. In a blender, blend the other ingredients. Pour the dressing over the greens.

Gorgeous Green Salad *by John Kohler*
Serves 2

assortment of leafy greens
2 pints cherry tomatoes
1 lg. avocado
1/2 cup orange juice

Blend 1 pint cherry tomatoes, 1/2 cup orange juice and 1/2 an avocado in a blender to make a creamy dressing. Arrange some of the whole leafy greens on the bottom of a salad bowl. Shred or finely slice the remaining greens, then place them on top of the whole leaves. Pour the dressing on top, then garnish with cherry tomatoes and long slices of avocado.

Fresh Summer Salad *by Christina Chadney*
Makes 2 salad-course servings, or 1 large main salad.

Salad
2 heads butter or red leaf lettuce, torn or chopped
1 punnet strawberries, sliced
1 punnet red or yellow cherry tomatoes, quartered
1 punnet raspberries, whole
2 or 3 sprigs of basil, shredded
2 or 3 sprigs of parsley, minced fine
optional: 1 English cucumber, quartered and thinly sliced

Dressing
juice of 2 oranges
1/2 avocado

Blend the dressing ingredients till smooth, dress the salad, serve and enjoy al fresco!

Sweet Spiralized Salad *by Cecilia Benjumea*
bell peppers
fennel
gold and red beets
carrots
cucumbers
summer and winter squash

Spiralize or julienne the foods of your choice and arrange them individually on a platter with a bowl placed in the middle. Fill the bowl with your favorite dressing, then garnish the platter with fennel stems.

Mango Salad *by Betsy De Gress*
Serves 2

4 ripe mangos, peeled and cubed
1/2 head romaine or leaf lettuce
1/2 bunch cilantro, chopped
1 sweet red bell pepper, diced
2 leaves of rinsed dulse, chopped
1 lemon, juiced

Wash and tear the lettuce and place in a salad bowl. To the salad bowl add 1/2 of the mango cubes, pepper, dulse and cilantro (scallions if desired). Blend remaining mango with lemon juice in a blender and pour over salad as dressing.

Broccoli & Bok Choy Salad *by Phyllis Avery*
Serves 2

Salad
broccoli florets
2 bok choy leaves and stems, cut lengthwise then slivered diagonally
2 med. tomatoes, chopped
1 cup sunflower sprout greens
1/3 cup chopped walnuts

Dressing
1 med. or sm. tomatillo
1/2 med. cucumber, chopped
1 lg. Haas avocado
1/4 to 1/2 tsp. dill
Cut the avocado in half, remove the pit and remove the pulp with a spoon.

Blend the tomatillo and cucumber. Add avocado, blending until creamy. Add dill to taste. Pour over the salad.

Spinach & Jerusalem Artichoke Salad *by Phyllis Avery*
Serves 2

2 bunches spinach
1/2 cup Jerusalem artichokes (sun chokes), scrubbed, grated
1 red pepper, diced
1 yellow pepper, diced
cucumber-avocado-dulse dressing

Remove the stems and tear the spinach. Combine the first 4 ingredients. Pour the dressing over the top.

Zucchini, Carrot & Avocado Salad *by Phyllis Avery*
Serves 2

2 med. zucchini, grated
1 lg. Haas avocado
1 lg. carrot, grated
salad greens

Grate the zucchini and carrot. Cut the avocado in half. Remove the pit and scoop out the flesh. Add to the zucchini and carrot and mix. Make a bed of greens. Spoon the mixture over the top.

Sprouts

Sunflower Greens *by Living Nutrition*
1 lb. or more of sunflower seeds in the shell
1 cafeteria tray
organic, non-sterile, sifted soil
paper sheets
water

Place dirt on tray and level it. Densely add sunflower seeds over the dirt, lightly pressing them down. Thoroughly water the seeds. Cover with paper sheets. Repeat watering every day. On the third day remove the paper and place the tray of sprouts in the sun, continuing the watering. Allow the sprouts to grow to a height of approx. 3 inches. The green leaves are tastiest during their initial growth phase. During their next growth phase a third leaf forms and the sprout becomes bitter—it's too late to eat them.

Dressings

Chunky Tomato Dressing *by Living Nutrition*
tomato, diced
sunflower, sesame or pumpkin seeds, soaked 12 hours, rinsed then germinated 12 hours, or, optionally, diced avocado
lemon or grapefruit juice to taste
basil or other herb to taste

Blend all ingredients except the tomato to a creamy consistency. Add the tomato and blend briefly to get a chunky texture.

Tomacado Dressing *by Living Nutrition*
1 sm. avocado
1 lg. tomato, diced
2 tsp. fresh lemon juice
2 to 4 celery stalks

Juice the celery stalks. Blend all ingredients in a bowl, adding celery juice to desired consistency.

Carrocado Dressing *by Living Nutrition*
4 to 6 carrots
1/2 avocado

Juice the carrots. Blend the carrot juice and avocado in a bowl or blender.

Cucado Dressing *by Living Nutrition*
1 lg. cucumber
1/2 sm. avocado
1/2 fennel bulb
1 tsp. lemon or pink grapefruit juice

Blend and serve.

Macadamia Delight Dressing *by Living Nutrition*

1/8-1/4 cup macadamia nuts
1 orange, juiced

Blend and serve.

Mint Tahini Dressing *by Susan Smith Jones, Ph.D.*

1 cup fresh mint leaves, chopped
1/4 cup raw sesame tahini
1/4 cup purified water
3 tbsp. fresh squeezed lemon juice

In a blender or food processor, blend all ingredients until smooth. Will remain fresh in the refrigerator for up to 5 days.

Minty Mango Dressing *by Cecilia Benjumea*

2 mangos, diced
1 lime, juiced
2 lg. or 4 sm. mint leaves

Blend all ingredients until smooth, adding mint to taste.

A-Maizing Dressing *by Betsy De Gress*

niblets from 3 or 4 ears of fresh sweet corn
2 sm. or 1 lg. avocado
1 cup cherry tomatoes
1 lemon, juiced
fresh basil to taste

Purée the tomatoes in a blender. Add the avocado, blending until smooth. Add the corn niblets, basil and lemon juice. Purée until creamy. Serve as a salad dressing or pour over an Italian dish.

Deep Green Salad Dressing *by Betsy De Gress*
1/2 cup tomato, cherry or heirloom
1/2 cup fresh parsley
1 stalk celery
1 sm. or med. red bell pepper
1/4 cup soft nuts (walnuts, pine nuts, pecans, or soaked almonds)
choice of crushed red pepper flakes, organic herbs, garlic, etc. per desired taste

In a blender, purée the tomato. Add celery and pepper then blend until smooth. Add nuts and parsley and blend until smooth. Add the flavorings of choice. Add more parsley or nuts as needed to thicken. Mix well into a garden salad.

Super Pecan Dressing or Dip *by Marti Wheeler*
3 to 4 tomatillos, or juice from a sm. lime
1 grapefruit, juiced
1/2 pt. cherry tomatoes
4 to 5 stalks of celery, diced
6 oz. shelled pecans

Remove the skins of the tomatillos. Add the skinned tomatillos (or lime juice) and tomatoes to a blender and blend until liquefied, then add some celery and continue to blend. Stop the blender and taste the mixture. If too sweet or acidic, add more celery to taste. When the desired taste is achieved, slowly blend in the pecans.

Sunflower Seed Dressing *by Katherine Dichter*
1 cup raw sunflower seeds
1/2 to 1 lemon, juiced
1 sm. handful of fresh basil or dill
1-1/2 cups water

Soak the sunflower seeds in purified water overnight, drain then rinse. Grind the seeds in a blender, slowly adding the water for desired consistency, then lemon juice, basil or dill.

Avocado-Tomato Dressing *by Phyllis Avery*
1 lg., tomato, chopped
1/2 med. cucumber, peeled, chopped
flesh from 1 sm. Haas avocado

Place all ingredients in a blender in the above order. Blend until smooth.

Creamy Celery Dressing *by Phyllis Avery*
1/2 med. cucumber, peeled, chopped
1 sm. pickling cucumber, chopped
3/4 cup celery, chopped
1/4 cup walnuts, ground

Add ingredients in the above order in a blender. Blend until creamy.

Creamy Cucumber Dressing *by Phyllis Avery*
juice from 1/2 pink grapefruit
1 med. cucumber, peeled and chopped
1/2 cup ground fresh walnuts

Blend until smooth.

Creamy Tomato Dressing *by Phyllis Avery*
2 cups tomatoes, chopped
1/4 cup dried tomatoes, soaked, drained, chopped
1/2 cup walnuts, ground
1 tbsp. dulse flakes

Blend until smooth.

Dips, Salsas & Spreads

Pistachio Salsa *by T. C. Fry*

Salsa
8 oz. of pistachios
2 lbs. of tomatoes, cherry tomatoes and/or others
4 tomatillos for a remarkable Mexican flavor
3 stalks of celery
2 red bell peppers

Platter Bed & Dippers
lettuce leaves
4 to 6 stalks of celery
2 cucumbers

Chop about 28 ounces of the tomatoes and add to a bowl. Add about 4 ounces of the tomatoes, preferably cherry, to a blender. Cut up and add the tomatillos to the blender. Blend the tomatoes and tomatillos, then add to the bowl with the cut tomatoes. Dice 3 stalks of celery and add to the bowl. Mix in the pistachios and stir well. Cut the red bell peppers into 2-inch pieces. Cut the remaining celery into 2 to 4-inch pieces. Slice the cucumbers. Spread the lettuce leaves over a plate or platter. Serve the salsa over the lettuce leaves, using the bell pepper and celery pieces as dippers.

Wholey Guacamole! *by Living Nutrition*
flesh from 2 ripe avocados
1/2 red bell pepper, sliced
1 tomato, sliced into chunks
niblets from 1 ear of fresh corn
1 tbsp. lime or lemon juice

Scoop the avocado flesh into a mixing bowl. Process the onion, bell pepper, tomato and celery, or finely chop with a knife. Include garlic if desired. Mash the avocado with a fork, blending in the processed ingredients, corn niblets and lime or lemon juice. Serve with veggie sticks and/or dehydrated veggie chips.

Nut & Seed Cheese *by Living Nutrition*
2 cups of choice of sunflower seeds, pumpkin seeds or squash kernels
optional: add or substitute 1 cup almonds
1 tbsp. fresh basil or dill, finely minced

1 tbsp. lemon juice

Soak the seeds and/or almonds together for 12 hours in a sprouting jar or a bowl. Rinse well, drain and allow to sprout for no more than 4 hours. Add all ingredients to a food processor and process to a fine consistency. Place the cheese in a bowl. Garnish as desired. Serve as a veggie stick, chip or cracker spread or dip, as a lettuce "handwich" filler or a pizza topping. Serve immediately or cover and refrigerate. Will keep in the refrigerator for approx. 24 hours.

Cucumber-Mango Salsa *by Cecilia Benjumea*
1 avocado, diced
1 bunch cilantro, coarsely chopped
1 English cucumber, diced
2 mangos, diced
1 lime, juiced

Blend and serve.

Seasonings

Lemon-Celery Seasoning *by Art Baker*
Forget salty, toxic, lifeless tamari, liquid aminos, namu shoyu, soy sauce, miso and other bottled seasonings and try this instead: dehydrated celery and lemon slices. As the celery dries out, it hardens and becomes thin floss. Cut the rind off the dehydrated lemon and discard. Place the celery and lemon in a coffee grinder and pulverize into powder. This is very salty, with a slight celery flavor, making it a great addition to guacamole, salsa, raw soups, raw crackers, etc.

Dehydrated Tomato Soak Water *by Living Nutrition*
Again, forget salty, toxic lifeless tamari, liquid aminos, namu shoyu, soy sauce, miso and other bottled seasonings. Dried tomato soak water makes a naturally salty and nontoxic seasoning. Soak dried tomatoes for 2 to 6 hours then drain off the water. Optional: add fresh lemon juice, fresh oregano, basil or other herbs to taste. Use the remaining tomato solids in another recipe. See Tomatochovies below.

Tomatochovies *by Living Nutrition*
Slice cherry tomatoes in half and dehydrate. Toss onto salads. Optional: soak dried tomatoes in water, drain, slice into small pieces. Or use diced fresh tomatoes for the salty zing you are going for.

Soups

Cucado Soup *by Katherine Dichter*
Serves 1

2 lg. cucumbers
1/2 avocado
1 tsp. lemon juice
1 tsp. fresh dill

Blend all ingredients and serve.

Spinach Soup *by Living Nutrition*
Blend spinach, tomatoes, lemon juice and avocado.

Entrées

Pepper-Corn Boats *by Living Nutrition*
Serves 4

2 or more fresh ears of corn
2 lg. red or yellow bell peppers
2 avocados, halved and pitted

Using a knife, slice the corn kernels off the cobs, collecting the kernels in a bowl. Cut the bell peppers in half, lengthwise, clean out the seeds, and remove the stems. Remove the flesh from the avocados and mix with the corn kernels in a bowl. Spoon the avocado-corn mixture onto the bell pepper halves and eat like a "handwich."

Carrocado Mash *by Living Nutrition*
Serves 1

6 lg. fresh carrots
1 med. ripe avocado
optional: 1 to 2 cups broccoli
optional: 1 oz. whole dulse leaf, rinsed
optional: 1 lg. red or yellow bell pepper

With the blank plate installed, run the carrots through a Champion juicer, collecting the juicy pulp in a bowl. Remove the flesh from the avocado and, using a fork, mash the avocado into the carrot pulp. Options: Run broccoli through a Champion juicer and add the juicy pulp into the carrot and mix. Add the dulse and chopped bell pepper to the mixture. Scoop out a bell pepper and stuff with the mixture.

Zucchini Linguini with Chunky Avocado Sauce *by Betsy De Gress*
Serves 1 or 2

1 lg. diameter zucchini
1 med. avocado
1 cup of 2 or 3 varieties of tomatoes (cherry and heirloom are best)
1 lg. red bell pepper
optional: 3 - 5 fresh basil leaves, finely chopped
optional: 1 tbsp. fresh lemon juice

Cut the zucchini into 3-inch chunks and use a Veggie Spiralizer to make linguini (see product description in the back of this book). Place the linguini in a serving bowl. Pit the avocado, scoop the flesh into a bowl, then mash with a fork until soft. Slice the tomatoes into small chunks. Core the bell pepper, then finely dice. Using a fork, mash the tomato, pepper, basil and lemon juice into the avocado. Spoon the mixture over the linguini and serve with a salad.

Simply Delicious Pasta *by Cecilia Benjumea*
Serves 2

2 med. or 4 sm. zucchinis, processed to "pasta" with a Veggie Spiralizer
2 lg. ripe red bell peppers, diced
1 lg. avocado
optional: 4 basil leaves chopped, 10 sliced cherry tomatoes, 1 bell pepper julienned and dulse flakes

First place the diced bell peppers in a blender, then add the avocado. Pulse the blender, then blend until creamy (for about 30 seconds in a high-powered blender). Arrange zucchini pasta on a plate, then pour the sauce over it. Garnish with chopped basil, bell pepper, cherry tomatoes and dulse flakes as desired.

Do you need variety? Creating new, simple, well-combined, raw food recipes can be delightfully fun as well as tantalizing to the taste buds! To get hundreds of delicious, properly-combined, simple raw food recipes, Living Nutrition offers the *Raw 'n Delish Vibrant Recipes* e-book. Tantalizing raw food recipe features are also included in the back issues of *Living Nutrition* magazine as well as *Vibrance* e-zine. See Appendix D for ordering information.

5
YOUR NEW HEALTHFUL
LIFESTYLE

5.1
WHAT TO EXPECT

It's up to those with C&C to do the work to heal and to preserve their health by maintaining the Natural Hygiene healthful living principles taught herein and in many other books and periodicals on the subject. This book gives the keys, teaching how the body's "operating system" was designed to work, that is, how to restore and maintain excellent health.

By setting the intention of continuous self-improvement with the goal of manifesting perfect, vibrant disease-free health, we can achieve our loftiest goals and never experience C&C again. Lifelong vibrant, disease-free health can be maintained by the daily diligent application of healthful living practices. The more we work at it, the easier it becomes. In time, it is no longer work; rather, it is automatic, pleasurable habit and the rewards are joyous. Deep down inside, this is what your bowel and your entire being is calling for! It's all about integrity—giving yourself the loving nurturance you need to be healthy. Taking care of yourself is always priority number one.

When you diligently apply the principles of healthful living, fulfilling the "Prime Requisites of Health" and obeying "The Laws of Life," you can expect ever-increasing wellness and joy in living. The further you progress with your healthful practices, the easier it becomes. Eventually it all becomes "first nature," that is, normal, sensible, effortless and enjoyable. Visualize a healthy mind, body and lifestyle. Think healthfully. Act healthfully. Live healthfully. In all ways be healthy. Claim your birthright to glorious health, allow the new healthy you to blossom and don't look back!

Health can be regained but it must be earned each and every day. Choose to live and be healthy every day. I encourage you to totally go for it, to dedicate three to six months to fully implement the self-healing protocol and get the help you need to see it through and keep up the healthful living practices. The reward is vibrant health, freedom and joy. You will love yourself, love life and derive immense pleasure in sharing your experience and high vitality with others.

If you experience some pitfalls—we all do, especially during the first few years—learn from your mistakes and keep moving forward. Becoming healthy and maintaining health is a lifelong process—we all have plenty to unlearn and overcome. Practice makes perfect! All successful people, regardless of their goals, work at self-improvement. The rewards of healthful living are all things that are truly good.

A Perfectly Healthy Bowel

Given the right conditions, care and time, if sufficient vitality exists, all inflammatory bowel disorders will heal under this program including colitis, ulcerative colitis, Crohn's disease, ileitis, irritable bowel syndrome, fistulas and hemorrhoids; strictures will also heal, scar tissue and polyps will slough off, tumors will be autolyzed and eliminated and the bowel will resume its normal shape with all new healthy cells.

When the bowel is perfectly healthy we are not aware of it at all! It does not give us any signs of distress and we feel free and strong. We have two or three brief, subtle urges to evacuate each day and the bowel movement is quick, effortless and in no way unpleasant. There is no more urgency, diarrhea, incontinence, constipation, cramping, spasming, aches or pains. As previously discussed, stools are moist, formed, have fine, homogeneous texture, uniform diameter, their color resembles that of recently eaten food, they have no odor or neutral odor, there is no mucous or blood, and they sink and crumble in the water. There is minimal need for toilet paper. We have little or no gas/flatulence and no foul body odors. With a healthy bowel we enjoy a sense that we are giving our precious body the care it needs, and we are rewarded with good feelings and dynamic energy, making life easy and pleasurable.

Special Care Requirements

During the first six to twelve months of rebuilding after the healing phase, the body still requires extra-special care. The bowel is tender and needs several months to totally regenerate the tissues and gain vigorous muscle tone. Eating a high-water-content diet, getting extra rest and sleep (10 or more hours is optimum) and conserving energy, rather than engaging in exhaustive exercise or work, is the prudent way to go during this phase. Conserve your precious vital energy so your body can use it for the rebuilding task—avoid doing anything (including fitness workouts) that exhausts your energy. If your illness was long and your vitality was severely vitiated (as in my case), be extra patient—expect the rejuvenation process to take a few years for completion. Although my colon healed quickly and my vitality continually increased every day thereafter, it took approximately five years to realize dynamic vitality and boundless energy after the long, debilitating illness and a lifetime of malnutrition. When I finally became dynamically healthy and fit, some people remarked that I was "the healthiest person they ever saw." After eight devastating years of disease, physical degeneration, chronic fatigue and misery, that was delightful to hear and it gave me even more reason to express my gratitude toward all of my mentors.

During the first six to twelve months, the nerves and tissues in your gut will be tender and sensitive to 1. excessive bulky fiber; 2. acids in acidic fruits; 3. excessive sulfurous foods; and 4. any putrefaction of high-protein foods. As such, avoid eating: large bulky salads with high-fiber content; whole nuts and seeds (they are best eaten blended with water or acid fruits as a dressing or in homogenized/butter form); large portions of citrus fruits, pineapples, nectarines and tomatoes; and excessive quantities of cruciferous vegetables, nuts, seeds and avocados. Thoroughly chew fibrous foods, select only the sweetest, ripest acid fruits and do not overeat. After your gut has fully rejuvenated, your sensitivity to fiber and acid will decrease; however, you must still eat within your system's handling capacity—you will always have limitations which must be respected.

Weight Loss

Expect and welcome weight loss as you detoxify on this health-building program—there is no avoiding it and the toxins and excess fat only keep you mired in sub-par health until you have totally cleaned out. As you lose weight, your body is working to clean out stores of harmful and useless debris, chemicals and excess fat. In order to totally heal C&C, all of the toxic and useless matter must be eliminated. Your body knows what it is doing and it will not get rid of anything it needs; it only does things perfectly and, under this plan, it will totally "clean house" and replace all cells with stronger and more vibrant ones, and will rebuild every bodily system for functioning in perfect health.

Many people resist the notion of detoxifying if it means losing muscle mass. Since the body needs an extraordinary proportion of its available energy for healing and rebuilding, we must relax into the process, abstain from bodybuilding exercises and accept these facts: 1. some muscle mass will temporarily be lost, but we mostly lose excess fat and water ; 2. the body does not need big, well-toned muscles during the healing phase and the first several months of the rejuvenation phase; 3. maintaining excessive muscle mass will only limit the energy supply available for the body's most crucial task which is healing; and 4. when the body has healed and detoxed and the level of vital energy is consistently high, it will be possible to regain as much healthy weight and muscle mass as desired—if you were a body builder, perhaps not as much mass as before, but you will certainly be able to fill out your frame and establish greater definition, strength and endurance in a cleaner, more attractive body than before. Understanding, patience and support are the keys to success—the payoff is the ultimate!

Weight Gain

Expect healthy, gradual weight gain after your body has completed the detox and healing. At this point, the body will automatically and naturally shift from the catabolic (breaking down) stage to the anabolic (building up) stage. Be patient and allow a year or more for the body to rebuild itself. To gain muscle mass it is necessary to exercise your muscles. Increase your exercise duration and intensity gradually. Do not force the rebuilding process by expending more energy than you can afford—it is better to rest during the first six months to allow your newly-gained energy to be used for regenerating your bowel tissues so that it can function at peak strength. If there is insufficient energy available for your bowel because of excessive exercising, it will not function well.

Building muscle mass is not all about protein but, rather, it is about working your muscles, getting sufficient recovery time (rest) and eating a nutritious, low-fat diet with caloric fuel content sufficient for growth. Calories from whole foods rich in simple carbohydrates are the superior fuel for muscle growth. In that regard, fruits, especially the calorie-dense ones (bananas, papayas, mangos, dates, oranges, etc.) are the perfect "building" foods, and they furnish adequate amino acids for protein synthesis. High-protein foods and supplements do not grow muscles—they only acidify the body, make it toxic and deplete our energy, sabotaging the rebuilding process and causing C&C. People with a history of C&C typically lose weight when eating more high-protein foods or supplements than they can digest. The diet espoused herein furnishes calories in proportions averaging 80% from carbohydrate, 10% from fat and 10% from protein. This has proven to be most healthful and sufficient for excellent muscle development and physical strength and energy for those with a history of C&C as well as all other humans. There are many world-class vegan athletes and a few fruitarian raw fooder athletes in the world who have proven this to be true; some of their stories have been covered in past issues of *Living Nutrition*.

By living healthfully, your weight will normalize at a level which is lower than the conventional norm, your waistline will be thin and your overall appearance will be leaner than others who eat a standard diet. You will also have a clean bowel and more energy for getting more out of life. Those of us who arrive at this condition are "normal" in true health terms. As such, it does not serve us to hold on to old images of our heavier selves. Welcome your new, lean, healthy body and cultivate it with the right exercise program for the strength, mass, definition and beauty you desire. When you feel great you will not yearn for the unhealthy bulk you may have been comfortable with.

Recurrence of Symptoms

In a small percentage of cases, several weeks or months after health has been regained, some experience a brief and relatively less intense recurrence of their former C&C symptoms. This is understandably alarming. However, it is best to remain calm, return to the simplest diet of juicy fruits and juices, get complete rest and extra sleep and allow your body to heal again. Recurrences of symptoms while people are strictly adhering to the post-healing diet plan is rare. The symptoms signify that the body has used the vital energy that has accrued from the healthful living program to enact a second "wave" or deeper level of detoxification. As such, it is best to appreciate the body's wisdom and let it complete the housecleaning. Following this second detox, you should feel better and function better than before. Depending on your condition of inner purity, it is possible to experience one or two more recurrences within the first year or two; however, this is very rare. Keep in mind that any future recurrence of symptoms must be scrutinized with regard to whether your diet and lifestyle simply exceeded your physical limitations.

During the first year or two of rebuilding, it is common to experience cycles of strong energy and fatigue. "Ups and downs" will occur while we are detoxifying and rejuvenating. Again, this occurs because the body has generated higher and higher levels of vital energy and this signifies that: 1. the body is performing deeper and deeper levels of detoxification and 2. it is allocating great amounts of energy toward the rebuilding of the entire body. Everyone experiences periods of tiredness while the body is rebuilding; therefore, we simply need to cooperate with nature, place our full faith in our health-restoration power, rest more and be patient with the process. In time your energy will maintain an even, high level.

If you stray very far from the healthful diet routine during the healing phase or even long after you have healed—even many years or decades later—you can, sooner or later, expect more acute suffering with C&C than before. Many have had to learn this painful lesson. To keep safe and well, learn the healthful living guidelines and be aware of but do not step into the pitfalls.

Emotional Sensitivity

As you detoxify physically, any suppressed emotional issues may come to the fore because the mind and body operate as an integrated whole. As such, you may experience old or recent familiar emotional feelings during the detox phase as your body releases old stores of toxins and emotional contractions. Most issues will typically arise and release easily. Some deep-rooted issues may be unsettling. It is best to approach the uncomfortable energy by allowing it to flow through the body for release without getting caught up in the memories and thoughts that arise. Simply bless the experiences and let them go. If the magnitude of any issues are persistent and too difficult for you to handle alone, hire a therapist who specializes in a somatic approach to personal transformation to safely guide you toward resolution and transcendence. At the same time, practice present-mindedness and explore meditation if that interests you.

Becoming more emotionally aware can be unsettling; however, it allows us to address our old "wounds," address some of the underlying issues of C&C and become more poised, mature, healthy and free. Welcome your emotional sensitivity—it's a wonderful gift which makes life richer and helps protect you from dangerous influences. By learning skills to master your mind and emotions, you will eventually be able to experience the world with ease and poise.

Amenorrhea

Amenorrhea, or cessation of the female menstrual period, may occur for a few cycles during the healing and initial rebuilding stage. This is rare but not uncommon, and it is not a cause for alarm. It is only temporary and it does not signify that monthly ovulation has ceased (unless you have truly reached natural menopause); females will still be fertile once per month. Amenorrhea signifies that the body has channeled its energy toward other more important tasks and, as such, there is insufficient energy available for menstruation. The period will return while following this healthful living program in one to several months, with lighter flow of shorter duration and no discomfort. This is another great benefit of establishing a purer body on a cleaner diet.

Pregnancy Considerations

It is essential to conserve energy during the rejuvenation phase following C&C. Pregnancy requires a great amount of energy for the growing baby. As such, a mother who has not fully rejuvenated after a bout with C&C needs to rest her body and avoid pregnancy for at least a year after beginning this program. This will allow time for vital energy to build up, for the colon to regenerate and for the body to detoxify, ensuring a healthy pregnancy for the mother and a healthy child. Rushing into a pregnancy too soon after C&C can debilitate the mother and lead to another bout with C&C.

If you begin this program while you are pregnant, continue with it and get as much extra rest as possible—this healthful living program is the best thing for mother and child and the quickest route to health. Breast feeding is recommended. If lactation flow is weak, try adding an extra ounce of avocado per day to the diet and, on other days, substitute nut or seed milk using two ounces of nuts or seeds.

Body Temperature

Expect to lose excess body fat which provided extra insulation against cold weather. If you live in a climate with cold winters, during the first few years you will feel colder than usual during cold weather. This is easily remedied by wearing heavier or more layers of clothing; placing a hot water bottle next to your body; sipping warm water; raising the thermostat on your heater; and preheating your bedding with an electric blanket. Keep your lower back warm at all times—dress warmly in cold weather. Never place an ice pack on your back or belly—this will tighten your spinal muscles and chill your bowel muscle, causing cramping and bowel dysfunction. By establishing and maintaining a good level of physical fitness via aerobic exercise, you will feel less sensitive to cold temperatures.

On this healthful diet, you will be free of the toxic load which overstimulated your immune system at all times. An overactive immune system raises body temperature and steals energy. As such, the standard 98.6 degree F body temperature is actually a "mini-fever." A purified, healthy body has a basal temperature two to four degrees lower than that of an unhealthy body subsisting on predominantly toxic, cooked foods. This is healthy and normal. It does not mean you will always feel cold or uncomfortable; it means you will feel better than before because you will be truly healthy.

Avoid eating cold foods and drinking cold beverages—room temperature is optimum. Also avoid eating excessive cooked foods—overeating cooked foods robs energy and cools the body after the short-lived warming effect has worn off.

During the day, eat sufficient amounts of the calorie-dense fruits (bananas, papayas, mangos, dates, raisins, etc.) which fuel the body, enabling it to create warming energy. Also, get extra sleep during the winter. And, if you live in a region with extremely cold winters and have a difficult time coping, make plans to relocate to a warmer region.

Dental Health

For many people, C&C and poor dental and gum health go hand-in-hand. The integrity of the teeth is largely determined by the overall quality of the diet and the acidity level of the saliva. Diets deficient in minerals, especially the trace minerals, promote weak tooth structures. Diets high in acid-forming foods are notorious for causing tooth decay and gum inflammation. A predominantly acid-forming diet causes the saliva to be acidic at all times, dissolving tooth enamel, causing decay of the dentin and eroding the gums. Negative, distressful thoughts and emotions also create acidity.

The answer is to eat a mineral-rich, highly alkalizing diet and cultivate mental-emotional poise. This will enable the body to detoxify acid wastes, alkalize the saliva, remineralize the remaining tooth structures and regenerate the gums to some extent. As you detoxify during the first year or so, the saliva can become more acidic, depending on your acid load level. This can cause further harm to the teeth. To monitor the situation you can obtain pH paper from a pharmacy or medical supply store and check your salivary pH several times per day. If your salivary pH is below 6.5 when you awaken and stays below 7.0 all day, this is cause for concern. Here are some methods you can employ to raise the pH in your mouth during the detox phase: rinse and softly brush your teeth often using water, or baking soda or a solution of sea salt water; floss daily; avoid all acid-forming foods; avoid all acidic fruits; avoid all oxalic acid-bearing vegetables; drink one or two glasses of fresh vegetable juice with dark leafy greens every afternoon. If the availability and quality of organic greens is sub-par where you live, you can try adding a spoonful of an organic barley grass powder to your vegetable or fruit juices—these powders are available from healthfood stores and by mail order; they are rich in a broad spectrum of alkalizing macro and trace minerals. When your salivary pH upon arising is close to 7.0 and it remains above 7.0 all day, your teeth and gums will become healthier.

Vitamin B$_{12}$

As previously discussed, vegans do not have a greater risk of vitamin B$_{12}$ deficiency than do meat eaters or any other people. People who have had C&C are prone to any and all vitamin deficiencies, including vitamin B$_{12}$. As such, it is prudent to have blood tests.

Standard blood tests for vitamin B$_{12}$ are unreliable. The most accurate test for vitamin B$_{12}$ is the urinary methylmalonic acid test (uMMA). The author offers the uMMA test through Norman Clinical Laboratory, Inc. in Cincinnati, Ohio. It simply requires a small urine sample, sent in a vial provided by the laboratory. If vitamin B$_{12}$ is very low, the level can be raised by supplementation. If the level is dangerously low, vitamin B$_{12}$ injections can raise the level. There are two common forms of B$_{12}$ supplement: methylcobalamin and cyanocobalamin. Methylcobalamin is recommended; cyanocobalamin contains a small amount of cyanide which is a toxin to be avoided.

Vitamin B$_{12}$ level will also naturally rise and, for some people, normalize via this healthful living program after inflammation has ceased. It is important to include some fresh, unwashed vegetables from organic gardens (preferably your own) in your regular diet. Vitamin B$_{12}$ is made by bacteria and left on the surfaces of plants and fruits. The trace mineral cobalt must be present in the soil. As such, it is prudent to amend garden soils and your compost with rock dust or other mineral powders which provide a broad spectrum of mineral elements. Unwashed produce is generally free of parasites when the local ecosystem is healthy, as promoted by good organic farming practices without the use of animal manures. When selecting unwashed produce, visually inspect the food for any signs of bugs or eggs—if you see any, it may be easy to wipe them off; if not, rinse the food or compost it and select cleaner food.

Health Freedom

Here are more major benefits you can expect as you refine and gain mastery with your healthful living practices, especially your eating habits:

You will no longer experience common maladies such as colds, fevers, gastric distress, candida, infections, headaches, earaches, rashes, PMS, difficult menstruation, bruising, fatigue, impotence, etc.

You will heal from or avoid common major diseases.

Your blood pressure and cholesterol levels will normalize. Your cholesterol level might rise during the initial stage of the detox as excess is dumped into the bloodstream; then it will fall.

Your taste buds will be delighted and never bored by the richness, vibrance, variety and complex flavors of fresh fruits and tender vegetables.

You will sense that fresh, organic feels more nourishing than other foods.

You will experience natural highs when eating tropical fruits.

You will relish and savor raw fatty foods more than fatty animal-derived foods and not miss them.

Calorie-dense fruits will warm and sustain you perfectly when you eat them in sufficient quantities.

Raw fruits and vegetables, eaten correctly, will no longer cause gastric distress and diarrhea.

Vegan foods will not make you tired and sleepy (unless you eat meals of mostly cooked foods).

As you become healthier, you will require less food to maintain your weight and energy level.

You will prefer simple, unprocessed whole fruit and vegetable meals.

You will mostly prefer mono meals of one kind of fruit.

You will require less sleep to wake up feeling refreshed.

Depression, unexplainable sadness, frustrations and moodiness will diminish and, in many cases, vanish for good.

Your ability to master your mind and emotions will become easier.

Your mental abilities including memory will become keener.

Your creative powers will become enhanced.

Your eating mastery and digestion will become easier if you maintain your fitness by exercising regularly.

Your waistline will become and remain slim.

Your skin and eyes will become clear and healthy looking.

Cellulite and cysts will vanish and moles will fade.

Your bones and nails will remineralize and become strong.

Your hair will become thicker and more lustrous, without excessive oiliness, thus requiring no shampoo.

If your hair was falling out, the rate will decrease after you have totally detoxified and, in some cases, new growth will ensue.

Your body will smell sweet or neutral, requiring no deodorants.

All of your senses will vivify.

You will feel richer sensations in your body

You will experience an expansion of awareness and consciousness.

Your eyesight will improve.

Your ears will become clear and your hearing will improve.

Your sinuses, throat and lungs will become clear and breathing will become freer and deeper. Your voice will become more resonant.

You will totally overcome allergies.

Your strength and stamina will improve.

Any chronic stiffness, aches and pains will diminish and, in most cases, vanish.

Your recovery and healing time following vigorous exercise and any injuries will be rapid.

Your medical bills and health insurance needs will diminish or become zero.

Your connection to nature, your spirit and your lovingness and lovability will increase.

You will enjoy the freedom of living under your body's own energy without relying on stimulants.

Your need for sleep will decrease after you are totally healthy.

You will wake up refreshed, clear-minded and full of inspiration.

Aging will greatly slow down and you will feel youthful.

You will look and feel 10 to 20 years younger than most others in your age group.

You will glow with inner happiness, knowing you have been "reborn."

You will gain a sense of being able to finally move toward your ultimate potential.

You will enjoy your new life and feel grateful for your new knowledge.

You will feel deeply satisfied knowing you are finally treating your body the way if was designed to be treated.

You will have more and deeper inner peace.

You feel more lovable and become more attractive to others.

When you arrive at the condition of peak health in a clean and fit body, you will feel natural euphoria and understand the true munificence of living in a healthy body.

5.2
HEALTH GUIDEPOSTS

Hopefully, this book is instilling a sense that health freedom, rejuvenation and inner peace are on the horizon. Embarking on a new, healthful lifestyle program can be an exhilarating experience. With Natural Hygiene as our "road map," we have the simple basic directions needed for a successful journey.

It's time to plan a new healthful life, one where you take best care of yourself so that you can enjoy superb disease-free health and happiness! Health is the result of healthful thoughts and habits. In order to manifest glorious health, we need to intend it, visualize it and put the plan into action with passion! Creating health typically involves a lot of letting go of old patterns which do not serve us and boldly stepping into seemingly uncharted waters. However, doing the "healthful thing" will feel right at a deep level, and that is what we need to abide by. The rewards for taking the best care of ourselves are glorious! Here are some key elements for designing a most healthful lifestyle. Take it one step at a time, be patient and good to yourself, and keep at it.

Dedicate at least three to six months to thorough rest so you can heal as soon as possible, rejuvenate and enjoy life in robust health. Complete rest is best; however, if you must continue working, do the the best you can—simplify your regular routine, work shorter hours, get help with chores and other responsibilities, rest as much as possible on weekends, take naps, go to sleep two hours earlier than usual and relax as much as possible. Conserve your energy so your body can utilize it for healing and rebuilding—avoid physical activities and social situations which stress and exhaust you. Remember: the more you rest, the more sustained energy you will have for doing all the things you want to do in your life without being limited by disease.

Key Healthful Living Guideposts

- Always eat fruit for breakfast and avoid fatty foods in the morning.
- Eat simply and lightly, keeping your energy level up mostly with fruit during the day.
- Stay fit and limber via appropriate exercise and stretching.
- Keep yourself well-rested and sleep-refreshed.
- Go 100% organic.
- Stay 100% vegan.
- Experiment—try new foods and become a "natural whole-foods gourmet."
- Don't overstock perishable foods—shop often.
- Buy your mainstays in bulk quantities.

• Frequent farmers' markets if available.

• When traveling, bring your own food and water, shop at natural food stores and minimize restaurant food.

• Go to juice bars and restaurants that have salad bars. Request plain baked potatoes, avocado and filtered or bottled water with lemon or lime.

• Plant a garden and orchard and add rock powder mineral amendment to your compost and soils so that you can enjoy your own fresh, nutritious food.

• Bring your healthful food with you to the workplace and when you travel.

• Associate with health-minded, supportive friends and family.

• Host vegan lunches, dinners and/or potlucks and have fun with them. See the Potlucks forum at www.livingnutrition.com/lnforum/index.php.

• If you own any of these, get rid of your microwave oven, barbecue stove, frying pans and coffee machines.

• Practice thinking healthful thoughts and reinforce healthful habits with consistent repetition.

• Medications do not maintain health and prevent disease—they are toxic, suppressing your life force, covering up your symptoms (which are valuable messengers!) and undermining your vital self-healing energies and health. Relying on your own self-healing power is the way to go!

• Go green! Discontinue using unnatural products. Shop for organic products and natural fiber clothing. Create a home with organic furnishings and accoutrements. Stop using plastic water and beverage bottles and food storage containers; use glass, ceramic, stainless steel and other non-reactive materials.

• Spend quiet time in Nature at least once per week.

• Take the time each day and evening to quietly reflect on your self-improvement process, and make plans to take further steps as needed.

• After you have healed, devote at least one day per week to total rest (sabbath).

• Think of your healthful diet and lifestyle as "normal." Conventional diets and lifestyles are unhealthful and common, but not in any way the normal human condition.

• Continue your education and reinforce the lessons you learn on a regular basis—that is the trait that successful people live by! Living Nutrition offers many natural health books and instructional videos. See Appendix D or www.livingnutrition.com/bookstore.html or call 1-877-740-6082 for information and orders. Living Nutrition Publications also publishes the paperback, *Your Natural Diet: Alive Raw Foods,* and *Living Nutrition* magazine and offers many other invaluable books on Natural Hygiene for educating and inspiring health lovers on their journey. Dr. Herbert M. Shelton's classic hygienic books—*Superior Nutrition; The Science and Fine Art of Natural Hygiene;* and *Fasting for Renewal of Life* — offer vital health lessons and are also highly recommended. These books have been most inspirational, instilling lifesaving wisdom for countless health enthusiasts, including the author of this book.

- Be good to yourself; lavish yourself with all things that are healthful—especially extra rest and sleep!

5·3
AVOID THE PITFALLS

Always follow the Post-Healing Vegan Diet Guidelines. The consequences of not abiding by them will, sooner or later, result in more disease and suffering. No—we can't get away with our former destructive dietary and other lifestyle habits! After all, we cannot violate the laws of life and get away with self-destructive habits!

Healing is not a cure for the effects of more abuse. We must always treat our bodies with special care, living within our biological limitations. Those of us with a history of C&C are forever sensitive—our body expresses "dis-ease" symptoms loud and clear when we poison its domain—and that is our great gift! Why is that a gift? It will keep you healthy and promote optimum longevity. Knowing your body's limitations is valuable. We are fragile, but we can be strong and enjoy a long, dynamically healthy life.

When we have not followed the guidelines or have not yet mastered our dietary and other lifestyle habits, we'll experience toxic bowels, as evidenced by foul stool and flatulence odors and other unpleasant body odors. If this persists chronically, our health will eventually go downhill: the bowel tissues will first become irritated and, as the toxic load builds up, this will escalate to inflammation and another bout of C&C. The only permanent "cure" for C&C is healthful living—we cannot get away with toxic habits!

If you should slide or fall off the healthful living path after you've regained your health, avoid getting caught up in sadness, sorrow, frustration or blame—get a good night's sleep and begin again. Instilling healthful habits takes a positive attitude and diligent, consistent repetition. Reinforce your lessons by rereading this book and some other Natural Hygiene literature, refine your habits and keep moving forward, day after day!

If you prematurely conclude that this healthful living regime "does not work," you have not understood the principles, have been misled by inaccurate beliefs, have not applied the healing protocol in a correct matter under professional guidance and, perhaps, have not given your body enough time to detoxify and rejuvenate. In any of those cases, an honest recognition of your need to learn more and think more deeply about these teachings can empower you to take the next prudent step toward getting the coaching you need to realize the health you desire. I and several other Hygienic Doctors are available to guide you to health and we'd love to help. Again, when humans correctly eat the original diet which they were designed for and take proper restful care, the inevitable results are healing and optimal health.

If you conclude that you cannot do this because "it's too hard," or you "got sicker," or did not get fast enough results, or you don't like the foods on the vegan diet plan, or you feel deprived and want to eat the foods which you are used to eating, please be assured that it's easier to be healthy than to struggle with illness and this lifestyle plan will work for you and you can do it, love it and exceed the expectations in regard to dietary satisfaction, energy and feelings of wellness if you give it more time. Don't allow your mind and impatience to defeat you! Letting go of self-limiting beliefs and working with a coach such as myself are the keys to success. I am sure you can do it because healthful living is your natural instinct and your deepest inner desire, and this health plan is the time-proven blueprint for success.

If you conclude that you need to eat some meat and do not want to be a slender vegan, be assured that meat and/or other fatty foods cause C&C and there is not one nutrient in meat or dairy foods which cannot be readily obtained in the low-fat vegan diet. Furthermore, the low-fat vegan diet is far more nutritious and truly satiating than any other diet and everyone can thrive on it, regardless of their initial mindset. If you cannot imagine this holding true for you, be flexible, give it time, read, contemplate and test it with an open mind. Many, like myself, have given up meat after eating it every day of their lives since childhood and not missed it at all, rejoicing over their renewed health.

If you conclude that you don't enjoy the flavors of fruit and are bored with the diet, or you believe there is too much sugar in this diet and fruit does not work for you, again, it will!—give it more time and be more resourceful. Fruit will digest perfectly and allow your bowels to function perfectly—in every case. After your body has cleaned out, your taste buds will come alive and be naturally drawn to the vibrant flavors of fruits as well as the fresh flavors of vegetables. Organic food will taste superior to commercial foods and you will feel nourished at a deeper and far more satisfying level than before. Fruit is nature's candy and everyone eventually concludes that there is no more satisfying food fare. The fruit-based, low-fat vegan vanquishes candida and blood sugar problems. If the quality and variety of fruits available to you are inadequate, be resourceful: drive to more distant food markets, order organic fresh and dried fruits by mail, grow your own and/or relocate to a place where you can obtain better food year-round. For more practical ideas on how to support your new lifestyle, read *Living Nutrition* magazine and get the coaching you need.

For anyone with a history of C&C, these are the major pitfalls to avoid, and they apply for the rest of your life:

• Eating too much fatty and high-protein foods—this is the #1 hazard (especially meats, fried and roasted foods), causing the most severe symptoms and worst suffering.

• Reluctance to take the rest and time needed to heal and fully rejuvenate.

- Eating haphazardly, without regard to food combining guidelines.
- Eating too much roughage.
- Eating irritating pseudo-foods, salt, spices and condiments.
- Eating too much cooked food and too little raw fruit.
- Eating too much processed foods.
- Overeating.
- Eating when not truly hungry, that is, when there is no need for more calories.
- Eating when you are not feeling well.
- Drinking alcoholic beverages.
- Succumbing to social pressures to eat and treat disease like everyone else.
- Ignoring "dis-ease" warning signals and not taking proper care.
- Ignoring the malodorous signs of bowel toxemia.
- Allowing the belly to become bloated with a backlog of food residue.
- Allowing the lower back and pelvis to become stiff.
- Lack of access to fresh, organically-grown foods.
- Placing your personal health as secondary to your family's needs.
- Impatience with the healing progress.
- Lack of sleep and rest.
- Misunderstanding detoxification and healing symptoms.
- Dissatisfaction with your low weight and assuming you need to stuff in more protein.
- Insufficient physical fitness.
- Insufficient healing and lifestyle support.
- Thinking of the vegan diet and lifestyle as "abnormal" or "radical."
- Disbelief of the nutritional adequacy of the Vegan Diet.
- Not knowing or believing in your self-healing powers.
- Not continuing your education in mind-body health.
- Believing that things outside of your domain (therapies such as medicines, acupuncture, homeopathy, colonics, herbs, supplements, etc.) can heal you. (They can only shift symptoms, enervate and fool you.)
- Accepting illness as your fate.
- Believing you can't do it.

You can do it! Every person I've worked with who at first believed he/she could not do it, later considered the entire healing plan more deeply and applied it, eventually succeeded. Believe in yourself and your magnificent self-healing power, the correctness of eating your natural biological diet, be wise, learn your lessons, choose to be healthy each and every day, plan out a totally healthful lifestyle and enjoy the process! The process begins with a vision, education, intention and passionate action. Visualize yourself doing it and claim your birthright to excellent health!

If you doubt the nutritional adequacy of the Vegan Diet, get your blood tested more than once—the proof will be revealed and it is typically stunningly wonderful. If your interest and dedication to healthful living fades, continue your education—study this book and many others from the Living Nutrition Bookstore.

Being truly healthy—feeling well and dynamically alive—is joyful. Health is our normal, natural state. You will discover this for yourself. Conversely, accepting illness is not the way you truly want to live. It takes a radical departure from conventional norms to heal and maintain the healthful lifestyle. Feel proud of your radical decision to become healthy the natural way–it's the only way and it results in happiness and freedom from C&C. With dedication, diligence and time you will feel awesomely healthy and be able to do more and get more out of life than you dreamed possible! Many people who've followed the healthful living path have experienced this and "kissed C&C good-bye." You can do it, too!

5.4
ABIDING BY YOUR GUIDING SENSE OF HEALTHFULNESS

Abiding by your guiding sense of healthfulness is the single most important skill for keeping healthy and living well. Your health, survival, quality of life and prospects of avoiding tragedy and suffering ultimately depend upon how well you obey this sense. With a bundle of insight tools in your pocket, you'll be enabled to skillfully follow the wisdom of your senses and become the master of your health destiny.

Providence has endowed you with magnificent sensory apparatus as well as an internal communication network which expresses vital information concerning your every bodily need. You can think of this network as the voices of your guardian angels, helping to keep you safe, alive and thriving.

No, I am not talking about New Age celestial beings, religious cherubs or other fanciful notions. I'm talking about the expressions of all of your senses which, as an integrated whole, actually serve as a guiding sense of healthfulness. Your mind is capable of abiding by the wisdom of this instinctual sense. And, with experience and skill, you can become the master of your health destiny.

The body is always patrolling its domain and talking to you, i.e., expressing its vital needs through the senses, such as when you are ailing or in danger. When you open up to this intelligence, you can access a fountain of perfect guiding wisdom.

Living successfully and maintaining superb health is not luck—it is your birthright, the outcome of appropriately responding to the messages of your body's inner wisdom. Truly successful people are proficient at following their senses, or focusing within. They use this information to make the right choices in life, and you can do this too. You possess the potential to successfully respond to all of life's challenges in all situations and create perfect health.

To become your own self-healthcare expert and stay free of C&C, you don't need a guru, a shaman, a doctor or a medicine man to tune in to these messages. You can become your own health guru or doctor via Natural Hygiene education and the practice of tuning inward.

The Revelation Of Disease Causation and Prudent Care

Via deep listening and an understanding of the basic principles of health as taught by Natural Hygiene, you will be able to ascertain the cause and solution to every one of your symptoms. There will be no mysteries concerning the whys and wherefores of your symptoms. You will know exactly why you became sick and will have the insight and confidence to give your body the precise nurturing it needs to quickly heal. You won't need to run to doctors—you'll know what to do! And you'll come to understand that the body heals best without interference, and gain the confidence to let it do so.

Tuning In

Tuning inward can come easily and naturally, or it may require work to develop this skill. At some point it might come as an existential epiphany or a mystical revelation, but it is neither New Age magic nor a religious miracle; it's a natural expansion of your sensory awareness.

To get there, some obstructions may need to be identified and cleared. We all have obstructions; they may be minor and subtle or they may be huge blocks. If needed, you might work with a skilled awareness development coach or therapist skilled in guiding people through the obstacles. When cleared, you'll feel freer, more comfortable with life's challenges, more expansive and more intuitive. With clear insight and confidence, you'll sense your inner and external environment and circumstances and know how best to proceed. Appropriate decisions with successful outcomes will come more easily and your health will have the chance to blossom.

Clarifying the Transmissions & Meanings

Unbeknownst to you, various factors may be limiting your reception of wisdom messages from within. In a manner of speaking, you may only be receiving a few fuzzy channels over a narrow band at slow speed. Fortunately, however, you do possess the ability to optimize your body "hardware" and tune inward and receive a "full deluxe broadband package" of all the vital messages.

When you are not receiving or understanding messages clearly, and perhaps having trouble making decisions, you can access clear guidance messages by slowing down, tuning in and patiently "listening," i.e., allowing information to bubble up to your conscious awareness. If the answers just do not come, your consciousness can be cleared and the messages made more resonant with a purifying, low-fat, natural live food diet, and/or fasting on water. Dr. Shelton's books on fasting will teach you why and how to fast, and there are a few fasting centers where you can get the professional guidance and comfort you need. The benefits of fasting include more clarity, keener senses, accelerated healing and overall rejuvenation.

At first, you may not understand the meaning of those inner messages, nor how to go about responding properly to them. However, you can become adept. It takes work. And, since your health depends upon it, it's worth the effort. After all, would you prefer to rely on sovereign health assurance or pin your hopes on the false promises of health insurance and the guesses and machinations of doctors?

No doctor knows your needs better than your own inner genius, and only your body can heal itself!

Awareness For Health & Dietary Mastery

Disease and health don't just happen—they are caused! In 99% of all disease issues our choices and habits are the culprits. You can change your health condition, even if your genetics are not perfect. You can improve your overall health in virtually every way via education and insight. Awareness is the key.

By making sensory awareness your moment-to-moment mindful experience, you'll be able to make decisions which keep you safe, comfortable and healthy. With regard to your health, you'll be enabled to make proper decisions such as: dressing properly to maintain comfortable body temperature; exercising at a safe level which prevents injury; resting and sleeping to promote optimum energy, performance and healing; sunning adequately and not to the point of injury; eating in a manner which keeps you well-nourished, i.e., hydrated, nutrified, energized as well as internally clean, balanced and joyful, and so on. More specifically with regard to diet, your guiding senses coupled with some life experience will give you the wisdom to precisely know: when you need to eat, drink and fast (rest); which food(s) to eat and drink; what quantities to ingest; and when to stop eating and drinking.

Freedom from disordered eating and other self-destructive habits is our birthright, and our senses will lead us there if we focus on the whole health process and keep at it. Knowing our needs frees us from confusion and fear, and we're enabled to reconnect to the natural order of life. When we are free, we are naturally dynamically energetic, creative, openhearted and compassionate toward all. This is the environment for creating vibrant health and keeping youthful vitality.

Self-reliant Health Freedom

By obtaining guidance from inside instead of relying on fixes from outside, you will have true health freedom. Your senses will faithfully protect and guide you, and no one, no doctor and no thing can do a better job of this. No one knows your health needs better than the health guide within you!

All of the finest gifts of life—peace, tranquility, joy and health—are yours. Listen deeply, get in touch with your inner powers, and enjoy the freedom!

Tools & Techniques For Honing Your Insight Skills

Becoming adept at sensing deeply and responding skillfully to wisdom messages from within takes practice. How to approach it? Try various angles as needed until the channels open up and come into tune. Here are some tools and techniques you can explore. You'll likely find a few favorites which will serve you well on your path.

• Think "natural," simplify and align your lifestyle with the ways of Mother Nature.

• Develop a lifestyle regimen of solely healthful practices.

• Do not accept stress in any area of your life.

• Become an observer of your body sensations, emotions and thoughts.

• Practice being present and aware at all times.

• Take walks, practicing awareness and presence.

• Know how your undisciplined mind thinks and disengage from unhealthful, inaccurate, disempowering health concepts, myths and deceptions.

• Find a quiet place, sit in silence and simply "be" with yourself each day, especially in the morning when you awaken and at night when you retire to bed.

• Go out into Nature on a regular basis and practice stillness.

• Tune inward, observe bodily sensations, energies, discomforts and other qualities.

• When uncomfortable feelings and emotions arise, stay present, accept them, disengage from the stories they bring into your mind, let the energy flow through your body, and release. Observe all of this from a neutral vantage point without getting caught up in any dramas.

• Become aware of your resistance to going deeper within. This resistance is exactly what you need to learn about, delve into deeply, befriend and move through.

• Take meditation classes and learn various meditation techniques.

• Take yoga and awareness movement classes such as tai chi and chi gong, and continue the practices at home and when you travel.

• If focusing within is a difficult concept, learn the focusing skill from the book *Focusing* by Eugene Gendlin.

• Communicate with yourself and others truthfully, clearly, meaningfully and with presence.

• Keep physically fit, emotionally poised and mentally in control.

• Clarify your windows of perception via a purifying, vegan diet of mostly fruit and, if necessary, fasting on water.

• Eat simply and within your digestive limits.

• Avoid excessive cooked foods and fatty foods (raw and cooked)—they cloud your clarity, dull your senses and inhibit your ability to access information from within.

• Honor your health needs by heeding your inner guide's direction toward what you need to do to maintain personal harmony, safety and health.

• Learn to say "yes" to your guiding sense and "no" to nonsense.

• Congregate with compassionate, sensitive people who also practice present-minded awareness and healthful living. Model healthy people who practice presence.

• Release fears—all of them—for it does not serve you to bring on any of them. Don't allow them to stifle your insight and your life. Your awareness will protect you from harm.

• Keep your nerve energy well-charged via securing adequate sleep. Sleep is the source of your daily nerve energy supply. This promotes vitality, poise, mental acuity and intuitive power.

• Accept "what is" and let it all flow. Your life won't fall apart; it will become more and more successful as you hone your ability to rely on your senses and just "be." Making the right choices and taking the best care of yourself will become automatic if you surrender to your perfect guiding sense of healthfulness.

5·5
The Art of Rejuvenation

Your Gift

You have a magnificent self-healing body—
you have it all.
Your body knows how to heal itself—
it is trying to do so now.
Give your body the proper care it needs—
allow your body to completely heal itself,
and it will.

1. Start With a Healing Vision

Move toward the picture and feeling of wellness.

• When you are ill, remember how it felt to be well, and remember how you looked when well.

• If you have never known wellness, understand that you inherited a body which was designed to feel, look and be well. It is your heritage, your birthright to feel, look and be well. Imagine the totally well you.

• In silent meditation, visualize your well self. Find an image of yourself living the wonderful illness-free life you've always desired. See the picture of your well self. With that, imagine the feeling of wellness in your body. Keep that image in your mind's eye and that feeling close to your heart and never let them go!

• Never allow anyone or anything to discourage you from fulfilling your vision of wellness. Believe in your healing vision. Believe in yourself. Say: "I am becoming well."

• Move toward your vision of wellness every day, and take full responsibility for seeing it through.

2. Apply the Principle of Natural Healing

Your body is a perfect self-healing organism.

• Your body knows how to heal itself—it is trying to heal right now. The instructions for self-healing are encoded in the genes in each of your body's cells. Trust your body's intelligence and allow it to heal.

• Your body is always communicating with you, sending you signals. Tune in and respond properly and you will set yourself free of illness and be able to totally rejuvenate.

• Healing is as easy as closing your eyes and sleeping. Your body heals most efficiently when you sleep and fast on water. Close your eyes every moment you can and allow your body to heal itself.

• Fast on water, or consume only fresh fruits and vegetables or their juices when you are ill. The digestion of heavy foods steals precious healing energy. Incomplete digestion contributes to illness.

• When awake, close your eyes, focus on the feelings of wellness and breathe gently and deeply. With the inhalation, bring thoughts and feelings of relaxation and wellness to those emotions and parts of your body which need healing. Exhale completely. Allow the feelings of relaxation and wellness to spread throughout your body, bringing new life with each breath.

• Every illness or disease sensation (or symptom) you experience is a sign that your body is working intelligently to detoxify, that is, to eliminate accumulations of poisonous matter so that it can heal. The uncomfortable sensations are signs of vigorous vitality and of rapid healing.

• It is essential to completely detoxify. Never suppress detoxification symptoms. Believe in your body's innate wisdom. Allow your body to detoxify and heal and you will become well.

• Get the proper professional hygienic healing guidance you need during your healing phase.

3. Eat Your Natural Biological Diet

Your body was designed to function in perfect wellness on a diet of mineral-rich, organically-grown fruits and vegetables.

• Anatomically, humans are frugivores. A diet of mostly fresh raw fruits and at least 75% uncooked vegan foods is the most healthful way to eat and the surest way to heal and rejuvenate. Eat simply—eat mostly fruit. Healthful food choices also include tasty raw vegetables, sprouts, and minimal amounts of raw or germinated nuts and seeds. Avoid nuts and seeds when ill. Eat no animal products. Fruit and vegetable juices are very beneficial for healing. Healthful steamed foods include vegetables, squash and tubers (potatoes).

• Eat consciously and only when calm and hungry. Exercise to create true hunger. Eating when you are not hungry or when fatigued leads to indigestion, sluggishness and illness. Fasting on water is prudent when there is no hunger—get proper professional guidance.

• To varying degrees, cooked food is harmful to your body and is the cause of virtually every illness. Heat destroys nutrients and makes food toxic. Cooked food poisons your body and clogs it up with sticky sludge, draining you of the energy you need for self-healing. Make a transition to eating all raw food—get guidance from a hygienically trained health professional to formulate a safe transition plan. Steamed vegetables and potatoes are the safest cooked foods.

• Eat fresh raw foods which taste delicious. Consume delicious fruit for breakfast and the most appealing raw foods later in the day, whole or juiced. Drink purified water as desired. Do not eat haphazardly; eat in accordance with the principles of proper food combining—this will promote complete digestion and wellness. Eat fruit only on an empty stomach. Do not mix protein foods or fats with starchy foods.

• Understand that food has no healing power—your body does ALL of the healing. Raw food gives your body the best raw materials it needs to detoxify, create energy and rebuild. Eat to live; don't live to eat!

4. Free Yourself of Energy-Draining Influences

Take full control of your lifestyle so that your self-healing energy is conserved.

• Replace incorrect beliefs about healing and nutrition with correct ones. The basic information is here. Continue your education.

• To heal and rejuvenate, you must fashion a new healthful lifestyle where your vital energies are kept strong. Avoid unpleasant activities and circumstances. Take the best care of yourself!

• Release worries and fears and cultivate personal power through education, emotional release and affirmation.

• Set up your home for healing and rejuvenation. Create peaceful living environments for sleeping and nurturing physical and artistic culture, including listening to and/or playing beautiful music and singing. Cultivate relaxation and serenity.

• Believe that you deserve a stress-free, easy life—you do! Say: "I deserve a stress-free, easy life and am taking action to create that now."

• If your life's needs are not presently being met, focus your thoughts on what you need and actively pursue what you need to be completely well. If you need certain comforts not seemingly available at this time, ask for them—there is healthful abundance awaiting you.

• Avoid air and noise pollution, electromagnetic radiation, unnatural toiletries, drugs, unnatural foods, and temperature extremes. Replace silver dental fillings with gold or nonmetallic fillings.

• Avoid non-health-minded people and unsupportive relationships. Associate only with loving, supportive friends and family.

• Enjoy Nature's refreshing beauty as often as you can. Take in sunshine, fresh air, flowering life and enjoy the companionship of loving friends and, if appropriate, pets each day. Live in harmony with Nature and you will become well. Say: "I am coming into harmony with Nature."

5. Exercise

The only way to build a better body is by exercising; only in response to increasing exercise will your body improve itself.

• Your body will not improve itself unless it is given a reason to do so. Your body needs to be active in an appropriate manner. The result of not exercising your body, not working your muscles, not stimulating your cardiovascular and endocrine systems, not giving your body the proper rest and nourishment it needs is physical and mental deterioration. However, your body has amazing rejuvenative ability.

• In order to rebuild your body, it is necessary to exercise regularly and increase the intensity and duration. Learn how to design an appropriate exercise program. If needed, obtain guidance from a physical therapist, a fitness trainer and a breath trainer. Chiropractic, massage, yoga, tai chi, chi gong, walking, jogging, hiking, bicycling and rollerblading are generally beneficial.

• Learn how to continue the rebuilding work at home and do the work each day. It is vital to establish a supple spine, mobilize each joint and free up any energy blockages via stretching, yoga and isometrics. Do not sit idle. On a soft rug, even while reading, you can gently flex your body and hold postures. Make your living room your "rejuvenation room."

• Exercise before breakfast and each meal. Do not eat when fatigued from exercise—you need to be energized in order to digest food. Keep your body well-hydrated with purified water, fresh juices and whole fruits and vegetables.

• Explore different exercises and sports. Do what is safe and enjoyable. Breathe fully and build up your endurance gradually. Observe your body's needs as it develops, and learn how to give it the proper care. Nurture your body and stay on the fitness path for life! Say: "I am becoming healthy and fit."

6. Cultivate Self-awareness

The continuous self-observation of your whole being and all of your circumstances will help you to make appropriate healthful choices in life.

• Self-awareness is the mentally-directed observation of the self by the self. This is achieved through the development of an internal witness which silently and without judgment observes the self in all of its sensations, feelings, emotions, thoughts, expressions, actions and circumstances. The goal is to be present or mindful at all times so that you can see your life clearly and become fully conscious.

• To develop your internal witness, sit still and in a detached manner observe every sensation, feeling and emotion related to your body, and every thought; allow all of them to arise and shift, come and go. Avoid getting caught up in the thoughts, or in judging or trying to fix anything. Practice this daily for at least twenty minutes, and take extra time when your are emotionally upset. Continue living with bodily and mindful awareness while in the midst of your life.

• In order to cultivate self-awareness, it is helpful to understand the different parts that comprise your whole being or self. You are a whole being made up of a physical body, an ego-personality complex (comprised of emotions, plus thoughts, memories and belief systems of the mind) and a spirit (also called the soul, essence, divine self, etc.). When you live with awareness attuned to your spiritual presence, you are able to live more lovingly, joyfully and healthfully.

• Allow and accept all emotions that arise. Deeply feel all of your emotions, for they are useful for your healing and well-being. Relax into your emotions and allow them to spread through your body and beyond. By letting go of resistance to feeling certain emotions, your self-healing energy and vitality will rise. Do not express emotions in ways that are harmful to you or others. Communicate mindfully.

• Focus your attention on your body and its needs will be revealed. Take the time each day to reflect on your observations, question all of your beliefs and revise your healing plan as needed. Say: "I am becoming aware of and am working toward fulfilling all of my health needs."

7. Be Passionate About Wellness

Express your healthful thoughts with emotion and they will become actualized.

• It is the intention behind your thoughts and expression that seeds the wellness you desire. It is the emotional force that you attach to your thoughts and your expression that catalyzes your healing and rejuvenation process. Think constructive healthful thoughts, choose to become completely well and be passionate about your healing process!

• What you think of yourself is what you are. What you desire to be is what you are becoming. Think about how well you are, how well you are becoming and how wonderful it is that you have the desire to overcome your illness and totally rejuvenate—appreciate yourself! Say: "I totally appreciate myself—I am doing my best and am doing a great job!"

• Smile, laugh, sing and cultivate self-accepting thoughts and feelings. Love your self-healing body. Love your whole self. Love all of life!

• Interact with other passionate, health-minded people, learn from them and share your passion and joy with them.

• Say out loud, with passion: "It is my highest intention to overcome illness and create everlasting wellness! I am taking action! I am becoming well and I am rejuvenating! I love this healing process! I am grateful for my whole life, for all of my friends, helpers and teachers and for all of the lessons I am learning! I completely love myself and all of life, and I am succeeding because I DESERVE THE VERY BEST OF IT ALL!" And you do! Yes, you do!

5.6
Healing Touch

All mammals instinctively give healing touch to comfort loved ones. Certainly, we all know the importance of loving touching, stroking, rubbing, massaging, hugging and kissing children, pets, friends, lovers and anyone for whom we feel affection. When accompanied by genuine caring and empathetic concern, touch works wonders!

Every disease condition has a corresponding muscular contraction. This is our natural response for protecting the traumatized area. The nerves in spastic, contracted muscles cause discomfort. In time, the contraction generally relaxes on its own, facilitating faster healing. In many cases, however, people consciously or subconsciously hang on to the memory of the trauma, causing the contraction (or "emotional armoring") to persist. This impedes the flow of vital healing energy, leading to more "dis-ease."

An effective psychological tool we can use once we've identified this pattern is to feel deeply the emotional discomfort in the body and be with it until there is a natural shift to equanimity (a resolution). When we focus our attention in this way, the emotional issues come to the forefront of our consciousness and can be acknowledged and released, transforming dis-ease to ease. Whenever we feel emotionally out of balance, it is prudent to become present and still and practice this self-help technique.

Additionally, we can employ physical healing touch techniques. For people recovering from illness, this can be essential for reconnecting healing energy to any traumatized and weakened areas of the self. Thus, we are repatterning and rebalancing the flow of our life force.

We can gently lay our own hands on our belly and become aware of the good feelings that arise, dwelling on and inviting the nurturing sensations to remain. Daily repetition of this practice can revive and infuse any body organ with new energy. We can also gently massage our own belly, kneading any tense spots to release the contractions.

We can also get the loving help of others and receive the healing energy which is waiting to fill us up. The healing energy of loving touch is the same whether we receive it from ourselves or from others, and it reconnects us to our whole, vital, natural state of wellness. In simplest terms, we are simply allowing the fullness of feeling the nurturing love within ourselves. The goal is to maintain that feeling throughout our body by maintaining whole, loving mind-body consciousness.

The Ancient Art of Laying On Of The Hands

Since the earliest times, "laying on of the hands" has been practiced by "healers" to aid the sick and evoke a healing response. Warm, radiant energy emanates from the vital life force flowing through all that lives. Every cell in our body possesses sensory intelligence that responds to this life energy. Various names for this energy include: "God," "chi" by the Chinese, "ki" by the Japanese, "prana" by Indians, "orgone energy" by Wilhelm Reich, "animal magnetism" by Anton Mesmer and "elan vital" by Henri Bergson. "Reiki" is the Japanese word for universal life energy.

The laying on of the hands is referred to on many occasions in both the *Old* and *New Testaments: Deuteronomy 34:9:* "And Joshua the son of Nun was full of the spirit of wisdom: for Moses had laid his hands upon him ..." *Acts 13:3:* "And when they had fasted and prayed and laid their hands on them, they sent them away." *Mark 16-17-19:* "And these signs shall follow them that believe; In my name shall they cast out devils; They shall speak with new tongues; They shall take up serpents; and if they drink any deadly thing, it shall not hurt them; They shall lay hands on the sick and they shall recover."

The Kabbala and the Veda healing system taught laying on of the hands. Jesus was renowned for healing people simply by the laying on of the hands. While it is often thought that the laying on of hands is a Biblical concept, it originated over 5000 years ago, in Chinese medicine, Ayurveda and many Shamanistic traditions, as well as other ancient religious and spiritual systems of mind-body-spirit healing.

In *Magneto-Therapy–The Laying on of Hands* (written in 1978) , Rev. Hanna Kroeger reported that laying on of the hands was known as a "royal art" which was mainly practiced in the Middle Ages by kings and other rulers. The kings of France's House of Burgandy were known as "Sons of Grace." Charles the Tenth was one of the most famous healers. He reportedly healed 120 people in one afternoon with the famous phrase: "The King touches you and God heals you." Kroger also stated that over centuries, "the sixth sense has developed in these people and is employed successfully to the good of mankind."

In *Wise Secrets of Aloha,* co-authored by Kahuna Harry, Uhane Jim and Garnette Arledge, the ancient tradition of "Lauilima" is described as a pooling of many hands, aimed at raising the lowered vibration of one experiencing disease. Lauilima is considered "grace receiving gratitude, an emotional safety net" that sustains wholeness, anchoring these qualities so the receiver never has to fall into lower vibrations. In essence, Lauilima guides people into the full vibration of love. Lauilima is considered to be the energy of God; the "healer" is simply channeling God's energy, or Divine intention, through his or her hands. The authors claim this yields "miraculous" results. Reiki is a similar ancient practice from the East that is usually practiced one-on-one.

The Mind-Body Connection

In the early half of the 19th Century, Dr. Wilhelm Reich's approach was to work with the body rather than the mind. The famed Viennese psychiatrist said: "It's not the psyche (mind), but the soma (body)." His groundbreaking work led some psychiatry schools to incorporate "somatics" into their approach and fostered "alternative healing" counseling therapies in this field.

In addition to or in lieu of attitudinal healing and counseling therapy, we can, of course, employ healing touch on our own and others' bodies. Loving healing touch can "re-mind" the body that it's OK to release the memory of the trauma and relax the contraction, restoring comfort and ease. Indeed, we can all use a parental or lover's pat on the back, or a hug to soothe the stress of life.

As Dr. Deepak Chopra said: "To promote the healing response, you must get past all the grosser levels of the body—cells, tissues, organs and systems—and arrive at a junction point between mind and matter, the point where consciousness actually starts to have an effect."

In his classic textbook *Somatic Technique* (written in 1991), Jim Dreaver, D.C. wrote:

"In the quantum, functional, *somatic* model, consciousness is everything. The practitioner is *partnered* with the patient. He is acting as a coach. He is teaching the patient, through touch, to become more aware of his body, focusing on guiding him to a more holistic relationship with it. He helps him become more *aware* of himself and the way he breathes, moves, holds tension, and so on. This enhanced awareness shows up as *presence.* The patient is more centered within himself, more grounded. He is *in* his body.

"Being present in this way allows the patient to have more control over his muscles so that he can bend, stretch, and move with more freedom and ease. He is able to align his own will and intention with his body's innate flow of intelligence. When the mind is not obstructing or fighting the cellular wisdom of the body through negative thinking and unconscious emotional and behavioral patterns—which is what tends to happen in people who are not grounded and at ease in their bodies—then the body's wisdom has room to operate and carry out the homeostatic and self-healing work it is meant to do."

The Advent of "Therapeutic Touch"

Modern-day scientists exploring mind-body healing, or "biotherapy," have delved into the laying on of hands. Dr. J. Robinson Verner made these observations on the experiments of Dr. A. D. Speransky, Director of the Department of Patho-physiology of the All-Union Institute of Experimental Medicine in Leningrad, Russia:

"Speransky's experiments have demonstrated to the nth degree that the nervous system plays the leading role in the phenomena of health and disease, and that infectious disease is no exception."

"When a child falls or hurts itself, it generally runs to the mother, who rubs the injured area, kisses, pets, talks to and sympathizes with the child, and soon the trouble is 'cured'. When a member of the family is sick, someone in the household (ideally) strokes the hands and arms of the ailing person, presses the head, rubs the back, pets the sufferer, and thus establishes a feeling of comfort and security. The 'healing hand' has been a by-word through the ages, and still is at the present time. The 'magnetic touch' is common parlance, and is probably as ancient as language itself. It is said that some 'inherit' this gift, and some are told that they possess 'marvelous hands for healing'."

Wrote Abne Eisenberg, D.C., Ph.D., a professor of communication: "The experienced...patient can usually differentiate between a pair of 'healing hands' from those that are not quite sure of what they are doing. Healing hands immediately establish a therapeutic rapport with the patient—a bonding based upon touch. Touch, together with reassuring verbal communication, has been found to not only have a tranquilizing effect, but also a definite healing power."

In *Reclaiming Our Health* (written in 1996), author John Robbins reported the pioneering efforts of a group of nurses led by Dora Kunz and New York University professor Dolores Kruger using a new form of laying on of hands called "Therapeutic Touch" which directs the healing force that is believed to radiate from all human beings. This process is conducted for 15 minutes, without making physical contact. Studies have demonstrated that it promotes pain reduction, relaxation, and healing results in a wide spectrum of illness conditions. To the dismay of some skeptical and pharmacologically-entrenched medical factions, Therapeutic Touch has been largely accepted as a treatment for burn victims and other patients, and tens of thousands of nurses in major medical centers, hospices and in-home assignments worldwide are reportedly incorporating this modality into their work. Skeptics would be hard pressed to dismiss its efficacy after reviewing testing procedures and reports of healing successes on numerous test subjects, including hospital patients. Given the AMA's attitudes, Robbins concludes his discourse on this subject by expressing the hope that the nurses don't get arrested "for practicing love without a license."

In other recent reports of incapacitated elderly people and patients who had undergone major medical treatments for life-threatening diseases, the health-promoting and life-extending benefits of gentle massage and of cat and dog companions (where, of course, petting and stroking is the norm) have confirmed our need for loving touch.

Quantum Touch, authored in 1999 by Richard Gordon, is reported to present a major breakthrough in the art of hands-on healing. This book teaches how to use special breathing and body focusing techniques to raise energy levels so that, with a light touch, posture spontaneously self-corrects as bones glide back into their correct alignment and pain ceases.

Belly Massage

Gentle massage, performed by yourself, a partner or a practitioner on your belly and lower back regions, can relax muscular tension, release pain, improve the flow of nerve energy to the colon and improve every aspect of its function. The keys are to be gentle and patient, avoid forcing, intuitively tune into your body's calls for attention, and relax into the session. Avoid belly massage if you are experiencing a flare-up of C&C and the experience is painful.

In *Unwinding the Belly – Healing with Gentle Touch,* co-authors Allison Post and Stephen Cavaliere assert that gently working the fingers in the area around one's navel is "the most powerful self-manipulation you can possibly do. It can be profoundly relaxing when done with gentle breathing, and it connects you to your center in a very real sense, starting a process that will immediately begin to release tension."

For rejuvenating the colon, one can use a technique of gently working the palms and fingers in circular motions around the belly. This can be performed on small areas of tension, in increasing spirals, or beginning around the entire belly. Massage your belly in a primarily circular, clockwise motion, corresponding to the direction of the colon's peristaltic wave motion. Visualize the peristaltic energy moving the colon's contents toward elimination, especially if your bowel is constipated. Breathe gently, rhythmically and as fully as is comfortable. Visualize release and vitality. Rest as needed and relax.

Delusional Placebos or Requisites of Health?

Are "healing touch" and "laying on of the hands" just palliative modalities which give temporary physical pain and emotional relief while fooling us into believing that our disease has been (to some extent) eradicated? They can be! If we were ailing and "feel better" for a while, is that really a healing effect? Not necessarily! Is it possible the touching or laying on of hands only waste our time and energy, interfering with true physiological healing? Yes, that is possible. After all, how can we be healed by anything other than our own mind-body wisdom (also called "Source" or "the God within")?

Our mind-body heals in its own inimitable way when the conditions of health are provided. Nothing external can heal us but, rather, certain external factors are requisite in self-healing. Can "healers" heal us? They can fulfill some of the requisites of self-healing, however, our mind-body does all of the healing.

Non-enervating, loving touch can indeed be of significant, health-promoting value if, and only if, ALL of the "essential factors of life" are incorporated into one's health regimen, i.e., if you correct any errant thinking and adopt a wholistic

Hygienic program with healthful living habits.

You must understand that the God within you actually does your healing, and you completely self-heal only when all of the conditions of health are provided and the body is able to complete its regenerative work. Certainly, receiving loving attention and touch do help the mind-body heal because they fulfill basic necessities of health, but healing is a process which takes time and consistent, wholistically healthful actions.

By all means, be good to your whole self and others. Give yourself permission to receive and give healing touch and to embrace life! The vibrations of compassion and love are resonant, spreading far and wide and deep.

5.7
SUNBATHING

The sun sustains all life on the Earth. It is the source of energy for all plants and, indirectly, for all animals and humans. "Take away the sunlight and all life on earth would soon perish. Deprived of sunlight, man loses physical vigor and strength and will develop a disinclination for activity," wrote Dr. Herbert M. Shelton.

Vitamin D is produced in the skin in response to exposure to ultraviolet radiation from natural sunlight. Sufficient levels of vitamin D are crucial for calcium absorption in the intestines. Without sufficient vitamin D, the body cannot absorb calcium. People with dark skin pigmentation may need 20 to 30 times as much exposure to sunlight as fair-skinned people to generate the same amount of vitamin D.

Sunbathing helps strengthen muscles. Dr. Zane Kime, the author of *Sunlight,* wrote: "Tuberculosis patients being treated by sunbathing have been observed to have well-developed muscles with very little fat, even though they have not exercised for months." He also reported that a study of the effects of sunlight on groups at a health resort showed that the group that was getting more sunshine with its exercise had improved almost twice as much as the group that avoided sunshine, as revealed by their electrocardiograms. Dr. Kime also wrote: "The Romans made use of the sun in training their gladiators, for they knew that sunlight seemed to strengthen and enlarge the muscles."

Cancer of the breast, prostate, reproductive organs and colon may be caused by not exposing these vital organs to the sun and air. Anything that blocks sunshine from penetrating the skin will reduce the amount of vitamin D that the body makes. *The Lancet* reported that people with lower levels of vitamin D are at greater risk for colon cancer.

Sunbathing does not cause cancer of the skin nor wrinkles nor drying of the skin in healthy people. Sunbathing helps heal us by building up the body's vital energies and increasing the oxygen in the tissues. Sunlight helps people overcome winter depression. Seasonal Affective Disorder (SAD) affects many people and develops into severe depression as daylight decreases in the winter.

Physical culturalist Bernarr McFadden wrote: "From the dawn of history the sun has been utilized specifically as an aid to restoration of health and as a means of maintaining and increasing it. The ancient Greeks and Romans, Egyptians and Assyrians, Arabians, Babylonians and Cretans, the Aztecs, the early Chinese and Japanese, the inhabitants of India and most other nations that were glorious in their day derived their superb health partly from their contact with the rays of the sun, and healed their ailments by their aid."

Hippocrates, "the Father of Medicine," practiced the "sun-cure" in the temple of Esculapius on the island of Cos in ancient Greece.

Dr. Herbert M. Shelton wrote: "In truth, man was designed by the Creator to enjoy the direct rays of the sun and the soothing, strengthening influence of the winds over the whole surface of the body. He is by nature a nude animal. A full sunbath in the nude is ideal. This is not a mere cosmetic measure, but a health requirement of greatest value."

Sunbathe every possible day for at least 15 minutes, exposing as much of your skin as possible. Observe your body's signals and discontinue the sunning when you sense discomfort. Sunbathing helps you in every possible way—enjoy it often!

5.8
EXERCISES

Appropriate exercise is essential—humans are designed to be physically active and the body will only improve itself when we exercise. Exercise promotes the rebuilding of the entire body with stronger cells, structures and organs; rehabilitation of neuromuscular systems; optimum digestion, metabolism, elimination and vitality; enhanced mental-emotional health; and joie de vivre. It is important to earn your calories by exercising before most meals if not every meal; eating when there is no need for caloric fuel causes enervation, metabolic imbalance, toxemia and, in some cases, unhealthy weight gain.

Conserve as much energy as possible during your healing phase, then gradually increase a safe level of exercise during your rejuvenation phase. Consult with your physician, chiropractor, physical therapist and/or fitness coach about devising a carefully personalized exercise program, read books on the subject, set up your home and lifestyle for incorporating enjoyable, healthful exercises and learn your limits. Do not work out vigorously during the first six months of your recovery following a long, debilitating bout with C&C—your body is not ready for that and, if weakened by excessive exercise, a relapse of C&C can occur.

Guided Revivification

With the physical pain and mental distress that accompany traumatic bowel symptoms, it is only to be expected that the vital flow of energy and good feelings in that area will be severely impeded. The diet and rest program taught in this book will greatly enhance the body's healing and functioning. However, if there are lingering functional difficulties, such as sluggish peristalsis, cramping, prolapses, strictures, pain, etc., some kind of mind-body "inner work" may be necessary to fully bring the bowel back to wholeness in all its "essential" aspects. As taught by the Diamond Approach and the Diamond Logos disciplines of mind-body spiritual development, these aspects include joy, love, serenity, clarity, warmth, strength and freedom. The goal of this inner work is to reconnect or bring "essence" back to the deficient areas in the body. (For further study, read *The Diamond Approach* by John Davis, as well as works by A. H. Almaas and Faisal Muqaddam.) When the mind-body consciousness in the bowel is fully infused with "essence," wholistic wellness will blossom.

Guided Revivification is a mind-body exercise for revivifying (or reenlivening) the disconnected qualities of "essence" within the gut. In other words, this helps bring back the loving feelings and vitality that have been overwhelmed by pain and lingering weakness. This exercise also helps develop your inner personal power center known as the "hara." Of course, this also means replacing negative thoughts about the bowel with loving messages.

Begin by sitting or lying down in silence and practicing the Somatic Inquiry taught in Section 4.14. Locate and sense any strong presences of good feelings in your body. Focus your awareness on the best feelings and delve into the qualities. If nothing comes up, that's OK--simply relax into the inquiry and let things be. You can try thinking of a most pleasant recent experience, such as a lover's kiss, a child's or pet's caress, a delicious meal, a warming sunbeam on your skin or another moment of joy. As you dwell on the memory, sense the good feelings that come up, locate the expressing area in your body, and focus on the feelings more deeply, allowing them to expand.

With your awareness focused on the good feelings, allow or gently invite them to spread toward a specific area in your gut which you sense is in need of nurturing. Gentle self-talk can help. Patiently allow the energy to move and fill up your belly with the good feelings. Breathe fully and become aware of how your belly feels as you allow the good energy to flow in any way it desires.

Focusing on the good feelings, stay with the process as long as you like. When you are ready to go on to another activity, retain awareness of the good feelings that infused your belly and affirm that you can continue to experience this at all times. By regularly repeating this exercise you'll be on your way to fully revivifying your bowel for optimal, lasting wellness. If desired, a trained Diamond Approach or Diamond Logos teacher can assist you with private sessions. For referral lists, see www.ridhwan.org/school/teachers.html and www.diamondlogos.com/index2.htm.

Healing Breath

As previously stated, when we breathe correctly the belly expands on the inhale and falls to a relaxed, neutral position during the exhale. Deep, full, rhythmic breathing promotes smooth, energetic peristaltic motion and overall wellness. It behooves those who do not breathe correctly or fully and those with enervated bowels to practice breathing exercises. My colleague, Mike White of www.breathing.com, offers literature, CDs and personal coaching for developing optimal breathing.

A basic exercise which is most beneficial for reinvigorating the digestive organs and the bowel and for promoting optimum energy and well-being is what I call the "ovular body breath." It is best practiced at least once per day, in the morning when you are still in bed, as follows:

1. Lie on your back on a soft surface such as your bed. (You can also perform this while sitting up; however, this posture is not as effective.)

2. Observe your breathing. Is your breathing full, moderate or shallow? Is your belly rising with the inhale and falling with the exhale?

3. Blow your nose if you need to clear your sinuses.

4. With your mouth closed, gently and gradually breathe more deeply and fully, expanding your belly all the way down to your groin.

5. At the end of the inhale, let the breath go—do nothing as the expansion naturally falls away; do not force your abdominal muscles to contract.

6. When the time is right, gently begin another inhale-exhale cycle and keep it going in a relaxed, smooth, rhythmic manner.

7. After a few breath cycles, when you are comfortable, begin envisioning and feeling the breath energy move as a pleasurable breeze or current which travels in a smooth, continuous, oval-shaped path beginning with the inhale at your nose, traveling down the top of your chest then belly, then curving downward on the exhale at your groin and traveling up your back along your spine, then curving around your head to your nose to begin another smooth cycle.

8. Gently continue the ovular breath cycle as long as you like. The more you practice it, the more it will become a lasting, involuntary, automatic habit.

The following more advanced (yogic) version of the "ovular body breath" exercise helps to further tone the abdominal muscles, bowels and anal sphincter, promoting greater control of the defecation reflex. Repeat the basic "ovular body breath" with this variation:

At the end of the inhale cycle, as the breath falls away and the exhale begins at the groin, gently and gradually tighten or pull in your belly muscles and tighten your anal sphincter to a comfortable level, then gradually release those muscles as the exhale cycles up through your head. Continue this exercise only if it is comfortable. As your rejuvenation progresses, your will develop stronger control of your abdominal and sphincter muscles and have effortless, more complete evacuation.

Stretching and Yoga

It is important to loosen and keep every joint, sinew and muscle in the body flexible, strong and free. Stretching and yoga can help with those goals and straighten a misaligned spine. Many people, such as myself, have overcome scoliosis, disc problems, headaches, joint pains, pinched nerves and chronic spinal subluxations and pain this way. For those with a history of C&C it is especially critical to keep their lower body limber. When the muscles and tendons of the lower spine, pelvis, thighs and hamstrings are stiff, the bowel is typically unable to eliminate wastes efficiently, causing constipation and toxemia. Avoid living with chronic stiffness. The goal is to maintain the full range of motion to promote optimum nerve energy flow to the bowel. Stretching can work wonders for relieving constipation.

Avoid stretching beyond your body's limits. To learn how to safely stretch, practice yoga and hold inverted postures, read books on the subject and also consult a physical therapist, chiropractor and/or yoga instructor, especially if you are in debilitated physical shape with brittle bones, extreme joint stiffness and inelastic tendons and ligaments.

A regular practice—at least every morning—of stretching and/or yoga helps to develop flexibility and muscular strength. Always stretch gradually and gently, holding the pose for at least ten seconds. Do not attempt to stretch if you are cold—allow your body to warm up. Always stretch before exercising, stretch symmetrically with respect to the left and right sides of your body and stretch and hold postures in positions which improve your posture and mobilize your joints without pinching nerves while breathing fully. If you are very stiff and stretching is not comfortable, try some massage, shiatsu or other body work sessions. Avoid massage with lotions and oils—they are absorbed into the body, clogging the pores, overloading the lymph and causing enervation.

If you have a stiff lower back, here are two stretches you can try:

1. Lower spine stretch: Squat on the floor, balancing your buttocks on the back of your heels. Allow your hands to either hang by your sides or place them upon your thighs. Straighten your spine, raise your neck, lower your shoulders and pull your buttocks downward, stretching your lower back. Hold the position as long as is comfortable.

2. Sit on the floor with your back straight and your legs crossed and folded so that your heels are close to your hips. Place your hands on your sides just above your hips. Tilt your torso to the right, going slightly beyond the first point of resistance. Hold the pose then repeat with the left side. Continue the exercise as desired from one side to the other, each time going slightly further with the stretch. If you feel any pain, stop and consult a chiropractor or physical therapist.

If you have stiff thighs or hamstring tendons, here are two stretches you can try:

1. Stand upright approximately three feet in front of a wall. Place your right hand upward against the wall. Place your left hand on your left hip. Position your left foot halfway between the wall and your lower body. Stretch your lower leg downward until you feel the back of your thigh stretching. Hold the pose as long as is comfortable. Slowly release the pose then repeat for the other leg.

2. Sit on the floor with your back straight and your legs straight forward. Fold your left leg over your right thigh just above the knee. Place your left hand on your left knee and your right hand on top of your right ankle. Tilt your upper body forward, stretching the hamstring tendons, then holding the position as long as is comfortable. Slowly release the pose, then repeat for the other leg.

If you have a stiff pelvis and hips, here are two stretches to try:

1. Sit on the floor with your back straight. With the soles of your feet pressed together, place your hands around the ends of your feet and gently pull them along the floor toward your groin. As your heels approach your groin, notice the stretching sensation in your hip and pelvic muscles. Hold the pose as long as is comfortable, then slowly release it. Repeat as desired.

2. Sit on the floor with your back straight and your left leg folded over your

right thigh. Grab your left foot with your left hand. Tilt your torso to the right and extend your right arm straight out to the right, resting it on the floor. Feel the pulling sensation in your left hip. Stretch slightly beyond the first point of resistance. Hold the pose as long as is comfortable, then slowly release it. Reverse your leg fold position, then repeat the exercise for the other side.

As you increase your stretching or yoga routine, your range of motion will increase, your sinews and muscles will elongate and strengthen and you will feel more energetic, poised and at ease in your body. Flexibility also releases emotional contractions and pain and allows life's stresses to flow more readily and leave your body.

Most if not all people with histories of bowel dysfunction have disfigured, prolapsed colons, impinging on the peristaltic wave motion and causing difficult and incomplete evacuation. The colon's normal shape is maintained by nerve energy and soft tissue connections. Enervated colons typically lose their shape and slip downward. Under this healthful living program the vital energy flow to the colon will increase, however, the colon may not readily resume its normal position and shape without the practice of inverted postures.

Inverted postures can be practiced in several ways. Always perform them on an empty stomach and breathe fully. Do not attempt them if you experience pain or faintness. Get help as needed with these methods:

1. Using a slant board (the easiest approach): Relatively inexpensive, it can be obtained from yoga and physical therapy equipment suppliers.

2. Using an inversion machine: These typically cost several hundred dollars. Some chiropractors, physical therapists and fitness centers have them. With your legs wedged around a padded support, you lean forward and gravity gently turns your body upside down.

3. Without equipment:

   A. At the base of a wall, pile pillows approximately 12 to 24 inches high on your bed or floor. Carefully use your elbows to prop your buttocks on top of the pillows with your legs pointing upward and your feet resting as high as possible on the wall so that your body, from shoulders to toes, is at a straight, inclined angle. Hold the posture as long as is comfortable. Avoid harming your neck—place a thin pillow or folded towel underneath it.

   B. Handstand: At the base of a wall, raise your body upward using your arms.

4. Using gravity boots (the most difficult and risky approach): These are available from some fitness equipment stores. The padded boots clamp onto the ankles. Under your own power, or with the help of an assistant, grasp a sturdy crossbar above your head, raise your ankles and hook the boots onto the bar, release your handhold and hang upside down.

While in an inverted position, you can try the following yogic technique to assist the downward (reversed) movement of the colon: Fully inhale, expanding your belly. Then take a full, extra-long exhale, allowing your belly to fall. Before you inhale, gently pull in your belly muscles as far as is comfortable while holding your breath. You will feel a gentle downward tugging on your intestines as a vacuum is created in the space between the diaphragm and the bowel cavity. When you need to breathe, release your belly muscles and take a full inhale. If comfortable, repeat as desired. Notice how your gut feels after you leave the inverted position. You can try this exercise again when you experience mild bowel discomfort; however, do not attempt it if your stomach contains food or liquid or if you are experiencing heightened physical distress.

Walking

Walking is the simplest and generally best exercise for beginning rehabilitation after illness. Walks and hikes are wonderfully beneficial for oxygenating the system, toning the leg and pelvic muscles and enhancing lymph flow, peristalsis, elimination, energy production, stamina, appetite and mental-emotional health.

Taking walks before each meal, especially breakfast, is an excellent way to enhance your entire day. If you walk after a meal, wait at least one-half hour.

Walking can be done at a leisurely pace or briskly ("power walking"). Stretch first as needed. Do not take exhaustive walks. Walking is best done in a natural unpolluted setting, for example: woods, countryside, beach, a park, etc. Bring a companion and a light backpack with some water and fresh or dried fruit as desired. Breathe fully, be aware of your body, disengage from mind chatter and enjoy the good feelings.

Jogging and Running

When you are ready to go beyond simple walking, jogging is perhaps the next best form of exercise for enhancing bowel health and overall fitness. If you are in very good physical condition, you may choose to go straight into running. Consult with a physical therapist, chiropractor or fitness trainer as needed. Obtain durable, comfortable running sneakers. Always stretch and warm up first. Avoid polluted air and exhaustive jogs or runs during the initial few months of recovery from C&C. Be aware of your body and the terrain and breathe fully and easily.

Rehydrate yourself as needed with purified water, juicy fruits, celery and/or fresh-made "natural sports drinks," such as apple-celery juice, grape-celery juice, banana-water smoothies, banana-celery juice smoothies. Avoid bottled commercial sports drinks—essentially comprised of sugar, salt, chemical dyes and water, they are toxic and of poor nutritional value.

Allow plenty of recovery time for energy restoration and the growth of new, stronger cells.

Bodybuilding

The body builds larger and stronger muscles and bones in response to weight-bearing exercise when it has sufficient nutritional input and energy. As previously stated, the vegan diet taught herein furnishes superior nutrition, including adequate amounts of calories and the amino acids needed for protein synthesis for muscle growth.

Consult with a physical therapist, chiropractor or fitness trainer before beginning a bodybuilding program if you are in a weakened condition and unsure of how to proceed. Again, do not work out vigorously during the first six months of your recovery following a long, debilitating bout with C&C—if you become weakened by excessive exercise, a relapse of C&C can occur.

Begin your program slowly; do not work out with weights every day. Keep your practices safe and avoid becoming impatient and rushing—look at your rebuilding program as a long-term project that yields ever-increasing rewards. Warm up and stretch before bodybuilding workouts. Breathe fully and avoid straining your body beyond its limits. Avoid exercises which stiffen your lower back. Most people with a history of C&C must avoid sit-ups or ab crunches because they tighten the belly muscles and can cause bowel sluggishness and cramping.

Following workouts, allow plenty of recovery time for energy restoration and new, stronger cell growth—get sufficient rest and sleep.

Push-ups are a simple, effective exercise for building up the chest, shoulders and neck. Perform push-ups with or without your knees supporting your lower body. Inhale as you push up and exhale as your body falls down.

Pull-ups are also effective for building the upper body. Sports fitness stores sell pull-up bars which can be mounted in a doorway. By hanging from the bar you can loosen up stiff vertebrae and straighten spinal misalignments.

Isometrics are also simple and very beneficial for strengthening and elongating the muscles and sinews, mobilizing stiff joints and improving posture. Isometric exercises work a group of muscles against another group of muscles or a fixed object. Inexpensive isometric rubber, resistance bands (or tubes) can be obtained from sports fitness stores. By pulling against the resistance, they can be used in various ways to work many groups of muscles. Bands usually come with instructions for many exercises. The bands can be tensioned between your arms, your arms and legs, or your arms and stationary objects such as a doorknob, heavy furniture, sturdy hooks, bars and posts and trees. You can also use the bands against the resistance of a workout partner.

Dumbbells are also useful. Depending on your strength, begin with 3, 5, 7, 10 or 15 pound weights. Practice curls, arm rises and leg rises while keeping your back straight.

Likewise, bench weights are good. Begin at an easy weight level.

Bodybuilding machines using weights, bands and pneumatic resistance are also beneficial. They can be obtained from sports fitness equipment stores or used at fitness gyms and studios. Get the coaching you need.

Other Beneficial Exercises

These exercises are also healthful for the body, mind and spirit—explore new ones, keep them safe and enjoy your favorites: bicycling, roller blading, ice skating, hockey, basketball, baseball, softball, stickball, whiffleball, soccer, volleyball, badminton, ping-pong, tennis, squash, racquetball, swimming (in non-chlorinated pools), surfing, water and snow skiing and boarding, kayaking, canoeing, bowling, frisbee, aerobercise, rebounding, gymnastics, calisthenics, dancing, singing, chanting, vocal toning, tai chi, chi gong, pilates, gardening, climbing trees to pick fruit and (of course!) carrying groceries.

6
<u>INSPIRATION</u>

6.1

ARE YOU POSSESSED OF COURAGE?

by Dr. T. C. Fry

Perhaps you'll recall the refrain:

Dare to be a Daniel;
Dare to stand alone;
Dare to have a purpose clear;
Dare to make it known.

If within you resides even a modicum of courage, you'll rededicate yourself to being a modern Daniel. And you need not stand alone! Mutually we can create thousands, yea, millions of Daniels.

In you I'm sure is the spark of courage that will impel you to learn what is right for yourself and, with conviction and resolve, do what you should do.

You will set as your goal personal excellence in all matters. You will strive to help your fellow beings open their eyes to the beacon of Life Natural Hygiene that they too may lead their lives in ways of righteousness.

As a modern Daniel you will not yield to injurious temptation and importunity. You will set an example for your fellow beings. You will become a living testimonial to the joys of living life on the plane our biological heritage decrees.

Dare you be a Daniel? Do you dare to stand alone if need be? Do you have a purpose clear? Do you dare to make it known?

Become a Natural Hygienist in all that this implies. You'll grow in courage and dare to master yourself. And you'll win from your fellow beings the respect that being a Daniel deserves.

6.2
Don't Quit

Author Unknown

When things go wrong, as they sometimes will,
When the road you're trudging seems all uphill,
When the funds are low and the debts are high,
And you want to smile, but you have to sigh,
When care is pressing you down a bit—
Rest if you must, but don't you quit.

Life is queer with its twists and turns,
As every one of us sometimes learns,
And many a person turns about
When they might have won had they stuck it out.
Don't give up though the pace seems slow—
You may succeed with another blow.

Often the struggler has given up
When he might have captured the victor's cup;
And he learned too late
when the night came down,
How close he was to the golden crown.

Success is failure turned inside out—
So stick to the fight when you're hardest hit,
It's when things seem the worst that you mustn't quit.

6.3
THE FRUITS OF HEALING–
DR. DAVID KLEIN'S STORY ABOUT HIS
NATURAL HEALING OF
ULCERATIVE COLITIS

This story is dedicated to the many who suffer needlessly in the dark.

With eternal gratitude to my wellness mentor, Dr. T. C. Fry.

Introduction

This is a personal account of my dramatic natural healing of ulcerative colitis, which followed my unsuccessful run of the medical route. Ulcerative colitis is one of two common inflammatory bowel diseases (IBD); the other is Crohn's disease. The major symptoms of ulcerative colitis are generally inflammation and ulcerations in the colon, bowel dysfunction, abdominal pain and sometimes bleeding. IBD usually has a life-ruining effect, and prolonged suffering with it can result in colon cancer. By the Crohn's and Colitis Foundation's (CCFA) estimate, there are 1.5 million IBD sufferers in the United States and tens of millions more with irritable bowel syndrome.

During my eight-year consuming debacle with ulcerative colitis, I consulted seven gastroenterologists from Manhattan to Boston. They all offered ineffective and devitalizing medicines, attempted to raise my hopes by saying that some day research would find a medicinal cure, and advised me that there was no plausible therapy for ulcerative colitis other than medicine and surgery. That all added misery to my misery. In the eighth year of my debacle, my colon ravaged with ulcerations and my health in ruins, I was given two options: radical drug treatment or surgical removal of my colon.

To my great fortune, shortly after I was given those options I came to a clear understanding of the nature of my disease and I beheld an enlightening vision: on a natural diet of mostly fresh fruits and vegetables, the diet that my body and colon were designed for, I would be able to completely heal and build new health. I immediately applied that vision by divorcing myself from all medical intervention and beginning a raw, fruit-based diet. The result was rapid healing. And I have not only fully recovered but have gone on to build superior health.

Regaining my health was my only course; giving in to pressures to accept my illness and follow medical guidance violated my spiritual essence. It is sadly apparent that medical doctors attempt to solve biological problems with illogical technological solutions, an unnatural course that perpetuates human suffering.

So, I hope that my story can be a bridge to a higher plane of thought for the two million IBD sufferers, and others at risk, who are being kept in the dark in a place where I used to live that I call "Medicland."

Medicland

Medicland, the place where I used to live, is reminiscent of Flatland, the metaphorical land of limited thought in Edwin A. Abbott's classic of the same name. In Flatland, a thoughtful inhabitant's will to enlighten his country folk about a dimension of higher thought is repressed by his leaders' status quo complacency. For his ambition, the Flatlander is tragically branded a heretic and condemned to purgatory.

Health truth seekers in Medicland are similarly repressed. When most Mediclanders are ill, they go to the medical doctors who only offer them medicines, and then surgery if the medicines don't work. And the M.D. renounces the higher concept of self-healing as heresy. Unfortunately, Medicland is a real place, where disease and suffering are a way of life.

As an unwitting prisoner of Medicland, I endured ulcerative colitis for eight catastrophic years beginning in 1976, when I was 18. I am now completely free of disease, owing to the changes in thinking, diet and lifestyle I made at age 26, as I'll joyously explain below. However, I often wonder: If some caring person had told me, when I first became ill, about a higher dimension of thought where the truth about the body's natural ability to heal itself is revealed, might that have saved me from almost a decade of unnecessary hell? I believe so.

Diet-Mind-Body Connection

Many people have asked me, "Colitis, isn't that an emotional thing?" To that, I say emotions were part of it for me; but you have to look at the related role that diet plays. There is a diet-mind-body connection. The standard American diet (SAD) I was eating before and during my illness was incompatible with my physiology—it was mostly cooked, heavy in toxins, low in quality nutrients and low in fiber. The toxins were responsible for weakening my body's defense system, decreasing my vitality, unbalancing my brain chemistry and irritating and poisoning my colon tissue. The lack of nutrients did not adequately support my nervous system, which became weakened, increasingly eroding my ability to handle stress. The mushy, fiber-poor foods led my colon to become bound with compacted waste. Synergistically, those factors led to increasingly "dis-eased" emotions as my colon became enervated, then toxic, then irritated, then inflamed, then ulcerated. The healthful love that was once in my tummy was smothered by waste and contracted emotions. The workings of the disease process are a mystery to the medical establishment, even though this information has been known by natural hygienists and naturopaths for two centuries.

Early Lifestyle

I lived a very comfortable life growing up in suburban New Jersey. I was fun-loving yet serious and sensitive, very athletic and always fit, with keen interests in sports and rock music. Although I was usually inclined toward humor with friends and family, negative thoughts and language were also a way of life with me. As I grew into my mid-teens, I became increasingly individualistic, and at this time many social and societal issues began to evoke negative feelings inside me. In response to the appalling pollution I saw in New Jersey's industrialized areas, I decided to aim at a career in pollution control engineering. My parents, great providers, supported me in my career goals.

In my early high school years, I felt driven to bulk up my body to enhance my performance in sports, so I ate large meals of meat and potatoes, or pizza, or sub sandwiches. Junky snacks were also a regular part of my diet. During that time I experienced severe hayfever and sought relief through allergy desensitizing shots, a treatment that only gave me partial relief while adding more pollutants to my overloaded system. Still, I enjoyed high vitality at the time.

In an honors English class in my junior year in high school, I read two classics that influenced me to become an intense idealist: Henry David Thoreau's *Walden* and Ayn Rand's *The Fountainhead*. Socially, I did not mix well with most people after that, and internal conflicts grew. Part of me wanted to go to engineering school to learn how to solve the world's water pollution problems, while another part wanted to forsake college and go live in the wilderness.

Also during my junior year in high school, in addition to allergy symptoms, I began experiencing nervousness, which was very disturbing. I had gotten into a routine of eating barbecued meat and pizza almost every day. Yet, overall, I felt great and was achieving in school, and proceeding with my career goals. I was also, unknowingly, setting myself up for a big fall.

Manifestation of Disease

During the summer before my senior year in high school, my health began to change. One day I awoke feeling very drowsy. I expected to be back to normal soon, but that did not happen. Throughout the fall and into the winter, my vitality and mental functions gradually became duller and duller. In November, I was accepted to engineering school, yet I couldn't feel any joy because I was feeling as if I were embalmed. In December, my complexion turned pale, and I became fatigued after brief exercise. Depression also began to set in. As this all happened too gradually to signal any alarms, I did not mention it to anyone.

In January, I was feeling very run down. I finally became alarmed when I began to pass foul sulfurous gases from my bowels. Then came incessant diarrhea. I then revealed my problem to my parents, and we paid a visit to the family medical doctor. He prescribed Lomotil to stop the diarrhea and asked me if I was eating a "good" diet, to which I replied "yes."

After three weeks of little progress, the doctor scoped my colon and saw some inflammation. I also had a slight fever. I was then referred to a gastroenterologist who diagnosed my condition as ulcerative colitis, and arrangements were made to hospitalize me. I had just turned 18.

Medical Treatment

In the hospital I received drug treatment: Prednisone (a cortisone drug) and Azulfadine (sulfa). I was also put on and advised to maintain a low-residue (low-fiber) diet. After a week of drug treatment, my bowels were functioning better. But, I left the hospital with my life shattered. The medicines reduced the inflammation but, in the process, temporarily burned out my adrenal glands, leaving me feeling perilously weak. In combination with the other effects of the drugs, I was left with a mentally suffocated and "spacey" feeling. It was traumatic not being able to function as I wanted, looking ill, and having to face my friends in my sickly condition—and that was only the beginning.

Unwilling to let my health sidetrack my plans, as I had no understanding of what was going on and when the illness would end, I dragged myself through a five-year university engineering program and then worked three extremely stressful years as an environmental engineer. During that time period, I had one flare-up of symptoms after another. With each flare-up, the M.D. had me increase the drug maintenance dosages. As symptoms would subside, I would taper the dosages down. But it was obvious that the drugs were not solving my health problems.

Those years were fraught with anguish, frustration, depression, physical pain and frantic dashes to toilets. My social life crumbled as I was too miserable to face even my best friends, and my predicament was extremely distressful to my family. Most horrible of all was the stifling of my mental faculties.

During the last three years, I experienced endless inflammation and ulcerations, spasms, some bleeding and stomach "eruptions" with almost every meal. I had become a physical and emotional wreck. What was once a wonderful life had become a traumatic, dying hell.

Throughout all of this, I held a belligerent attitude toward the doctors I saw because they weren't helping me. They encouraged me to attend National Foundation for Ileitis and Colitis meetings, but I rejected the suggestion because I did not want to join a group to learn how to cope with my illness—I wanted to regain my health, and obviously they didn't have the answer.

Diet Angle

At the beginning of 1984, the eighth year of my debacle, commercials for bran cereals began to appear on television. This was the first diet-bowel health concept I had heard of. While it conflicted with the diet advice I was given, I tried adding some bran cereal to my SAD diet. This small change did not make any difference. When I asked one gastroenterologist what the current consensus was on diet and colitis, he told me that diet does not play a causative role in colitis and no dietary changes can help anyone overcome the illness.

But, intrigued by the diet angle, I sought help from an M.D. who is also a nutritionist, in Manhattan. Because of heavy traffic and a restroom stop at a gas station, I arrived 30 minutes late. I was given a lengthy form to fill out and handed it in only to be told that the doctor had left the building for lunch. Disappointed, I went home.

Next, I tried a nutritional consultant named Dr. Laurence Galant, a Doctor of Natural Hygiene, who was then based in Staten Island (and now in Florida). Natural Hygiene (literally defined as "the science of health") is a wholistic health system based on the laws of biology and physiology, and it teaches that the body will self-heal if the conditions of health are provided. Natural Hygiene teaches that our digestive physiology is designed and best suited for a diet of raw/uncooked fresh fruits and vegetables, and that we can be biologically classified as "frugivores." In the 20th century, Dr. Herbert Shelton, then T. C. Fry, were the key leaders of the Natural Hygiene movement. In the late 1980's, the book *Fit For Life* by Marilyn and Harvey Diamond began to popularize Natural Hygiene worldwide. Today, Natural Hygiene is taught by Dr. Robert Sniadach's School of Natural Hygiene, Dr. Paul Fanny's University of Natural Health, this author's *Living Nutrition* magazine as well as other "Hygiene" educators and literature. People have overcome virtually every medically diagnosed disease via the principles of Natural Hygiene and there are numerous living testimonies to back up its efficacy.

Dr. Galant pointed out that the medicines I was taking were not helping me. However, as I was entrenched in the medical establishment, I continued using them. Dr. Galant also suggested a diet plan of mostly raw food: fruits and vegetables. I believed such a diet of "rabbit and monkey food" would only make me lose weight and aggravate my colon. But, as this diet was apparently working for Dr. Galant, who appeared to be in excellent health, I considered it and studied his handout describing principles of proper food combining for optimal digestion.

Desperation

In the spring, my health was in shambles and I had to do something. So I quit working and agreed to a second hospital stay. At that time, I began to add raw fruit to my diet. It was bulky but felt nourishing. I had my mother "smuggle" bananas into my hospital room and secretly hid them in a cabinet so that the nurses and doctors would not see them. The cooked, bland meals the hospital dietitian planned came with meat or cereal, salt packets and sponge cake or gelatin desserts. More drug treatment had results similar to my first hospital stay: a temporary and debilitating "quick fix."

That summer, I resolved not to carry on with any future plans until I was completely healthy again. I was at home resting and had another flare-up. Under doctor's supervision, I increased the Azulfadine dosage and gave myself injections of ACTH gel in my thigh, hoping that the latest flare up would be my last. Yet, the same pattern continued: symptoms would subside, then I would taper the drug dosage down, but later I would have another heartbreaking flare-up. My abdomen was always achy and sore, and I was unable to go for a short walk without having to make a mad dash for a toilet.

Reflection

My time off from work gave me the chance to concentrate on my situation. One day I sat in my backyard admiring an industrious squirrel sprinting back and forth all day, storing acorns for the upcoming winter. Why, I wondered, was this little varmint so energetic and unfettered, while I was sitting around in misery with my guts rotting away? Suddenly, a light turned on in my mind: he was doing his natural thing and eating his natural food, but I was not. I began to think more deeply about the natural way of living and solving my health problem.

I considered going to Columbia University, where my brother was studying, and using the medical library to research colitis. I thought that maybe I could find the solution in some obscure biology book; obviously the doctors could not. I never made it to a medical library, but I began to browse through books in health food stores. The information in those books on the connection between diet and health all seemed so impossible.

In the late part of the summer I began to appreciate the value of cleaning up my diet, as Dr. Galant had suggested. I cut down on, then eliminated, red meat, ate healthier snacks, bought a juicer and began making fresh fruit and vegetable juices. Dr. Galant encouraged me to stop eating meat altogether, but I was not ready to give up chicken and fish. I also experimented with acidophilus (a freeze-dried intestinal bacteria product) and noticed an immediate improvement in my bowel function.

Turning point

In August, thin, pale, sickly, nervous and miserable, I had an appointment in Manhattan with a prominent gastroenterologist and I told him about the positive effect that the acidophilus was having. He was usually well-composed and supremely confident. However, with a brief look of fear, his eyes shifted to the side. He nervously said that my experience was an "aberration," and he then emotionally renounced all claims of acidophilus being beneficial as "bullshit." I was amazed—this M.D. lost his composure and was scared! This reinforced my feeling that I was on to something big!

The doctor then recommended that I schedule a colonoscopy to determine the full extent of the ulcerations in my colon. A colonoscopy is a procedure where a flexible fiber-optic cable is rectally inserted to view the entire length of the colon. As I was still seriously ill, I consented.

In early September, after one day on a liquid diet, I had the colonoscopy. While a doctor was peering into the fiber-optic scope, a nurse was compassionately holding my hand. She said, "I'll bet you're looking forward to eating a big juicy steak after this is over." When I replied that I didn't eat red meat anymore, she looked at me in mild shock.

A week later, I returned to get the prognosis. The gastroenterologist confirmed that there were advanced ulcerations throughout my colon. He gave me the big picture: I had been ill for eight years, conventional medicine was not helping, and there was statistical reason to expect cancer within four to six years if the colitis continued. So, he gave me two choices to consider:

1. I could try his new experimental drug, 6-mercaptopurine, which, he explained, knocks out the body's immune system, which he thought might be responsible for causing colitis. He explained that if he could prove that more than 50% of 1,000 test subjects responded well to the drug, then he would write up the results in the *New England Journal of Medicine,* hailing the drug a success. I asked: "If the drug knocks out the immune system, won't people get cancer?" He replied, "Surprisingly, no one has developed cancer from the drug."

2. If I elected not to try the drug, I should have surgery to remove my colon (a colostomy), "in order to get on with your life," as he put it. He said that a pouch could be configured from my small intestine and sewed onto my anus so that I could function as before. I asked about the downside of such surgery. He answered: "Some people have trouble with the stitches ripping out."

As I listened to and looked into the eyes of the doctor, a heavy decisive thought came into my mind: This guy is insane—a Frankenstein—and I have had it with this madness!

Wow, did I have a lot to think about during my ride home! An emotional storm began raging inside of me. For the first time I actually began to think critically about solving my health problem—a difficult task, considering how dulled my mind had become. I thought there had to be a sensible health solution out there, somewhere, and it definitely was not with that M.D. I saw the reality of there being no future for my going the medical route. With my body and spirit on the brink of an abyss, I knew it was time to think my way out of this now. By process of elimination, I suspected that the answer must be diet. So, back at home I delved into the Natural Hygiene literature. In retrospect, that conference was actually the turning point which helped me save my life.

The Healing Vision

A few days later, while browsing through books at a health food store, I came across one $2.95 paperback, the title of which I have forgotten. It contained one sentence which appeared to me in ten-foot tall letters: "SOME PEOPLE DO NOT EVER OVERCOME COLITIS UNTIL THEY STOP EATING MEAT." Seeing that in print was "it," the big clue! Home I went and phoned Dr. Galant. "You can do it," he encouraged me.

During the next few days I pondered my last barbecued chicken meal, throwing away the drugs and divorcing myself from the M.D.s. Then, one night, I was studying T. C. Fry's Natural Hygiene lessons, and I thought about the assertion that fruit is our most natural food and a vital part of the pathway to optimum health. Then I beheld a wondrously clear vision: Human beings, the preeminent and most elegant beings on this planet, could have only developed to such lofty stature on a diet of mostly sweet, luscious and pure fruit—not on the SAD garbage I had always eaten. I understood that if I had nothing but digested fruit in my bowels, then surely the poison that was making my colon sick would be displaced and my body would gratefully heal itself. I also envisioned that on a "fruitarian" diet my body would be able to totally purify itself, enabling me to ascend to my optimal state of being; all of my dreams would come to fruition if I ate my natural biological diet.

Emotionally and spiritually, I was soaring. I had found the Rosetta Stone: I AM A FRUITARIAN! I now was going to take full control of my destiny, and it would be only a matter of time until I regained my health. The next day I announced to my family that I was giving up meat and the drugs, and with their support, I began a three-day fresh-made-juice cleanse.

By the second day of the juice cleanse, the results told me that it was all going to happen as I understood it would. I was coming back to life! My senses became keener and keener. I was seeing vivid colors again. My tummy was beginning to feel soothed and happy. My energy was increasing. My mind was becoming clearer and clearer. And I was feeling younger and younger. Once again, I was feeling comfortable with my world and in love with life. My overflowing joy drove my family and friends crazy!

The Healing Process

Next, I plunged into the study of Natural Hygiene. Most important to my healing was my understanding the lesson that disease is a natural process that the body enacts to heal itself. In response to a toxic condition, the body displaces ease with disease (or "dis-ease") as it focuses its energies on elimination (or detoxification) and healing. Disease is, therefore, not a hideous "thing" that mysteriously makes us sick, the symptoms of which must be smothered with suppressant drugs. Disease is the process of healing (or "curing") and must be allowed to proceed, but the factors that caused the body to enact "dis-ease" must be removed. Colitis is a manifestation of the body's vigorous attempt to clean out the colon and heal the damaged tissue. As I followed the natural diet course, my body was able to gently detoxify, heal, and regain its ease—the condition of wellness or health.

By strictly adhering to the principles of proper food combining as taught by Dr. Shelton, my digestion improved dramatically, and I was able to enjoy eating again with no more gastric problems. I assumed a diet of about 90% fruit and 10% vegetables, nuts and seeds in order to detoxify and recover as quickly as possible. Fruit I found to be always satisfying, and it helped me more than any other food. Almost every day I made fresh fruit and vegetable juices, for I found their cleansing and nourishing properties to be invaluable. Years of stored toxic filth and drugs poured out of my body, making me feel much better. Foul bowel odors were replaced by no odors or sweet odors. My weight went down to 118 pounds, from what I consider to be my normal 134 pounds. I did not like being so light, but I felt much better and was comforted by the knowledge that I was going through a rapid healing process.

Within four to six weeks my colon "dis-ease" symptoms ceased, I sensed I was fully healed, and I fervently began rebuilding with support from Dr. Galant. Rejuvenated, I went backpacking on the Appalachian Trail the next spring. I hiked more than 100 miles with a 25-pound pack strapped around my gut—the same gut which only nine months earlier was too sore for me to even endure the mild pressure of a fastened pants-waist button. Then I took a trip, a sort of personal renaissance, to Europe and Israel. Sixteen months after beginning my recovery, I got back into engineering.

With the help of a fruit-based diet, including plenty of purified water, plus daily exercise, it took me about three years to totally detoxify. And it took about six years to resolve all of the myriad physical problems caused by my earlier lifestyle, stress and medicines. I believe my experience and observation of other fruit-eating people confirm that fruit is the ideal food for humans, and a fruit-based diet, including the non-sweet fruits (cucumbers, tomatoes, bell peppers and avocados) is a key to mastering one's life. I was inspired to learn that Leonardo da Vinci, Henry David Thoreau and Mahatma Gandhi were "fruitarians."

Rebuilding

Psychologically, I needed to make a lot of adjustments, considering all of the emotional trauma I endured, plus the fact that I was trying to integrate myself into the modern world on a diet our ancestors gave up before recorded history. However, I was lucky to have Dr. Galant as a resource. His practice expanded into hypnotherapy and neuro-linguistics. He recommended books by Richard Bandler and John Grinder, the co-founders of Neuro-Linguistic Programming, and a book by Anthony Robbins: *Unlimited Power.* These books gave me the tools I needed to get my head and colon straightened out. They taught me how our thoughts and internal communication affect our health. Thus, I began to change my thought processes, and I ceased my old pattern of holding emotional conflicts in my gut. Using positive thinking and adopting a "let it flow" attitude accelerated my recovery and lifted me to a higher quality of life.

My posture was another calamity that I went to work on. I had severe sciatica, neck pain and stiffness. I went to a chiropractor who took X-rays that showed a prolonged spur in a lumbar vertebra, appreciable scoliosis in my upper and lower back, and a neck so misaligned that he asked me if I had been in a car accident. X-rays also revealed that 50% of my bone calcium was missing! Stress, malnutrition and other poor living habits were the actual culprits. In the second year of my rebuilding, influenced by the *Yoga Journal,* I began a rigorous stretching and reposturing program. It took me about six years to loosen up my spine to the point where I do not need chiropractic adjustments to relieve discomfort any more. Now my posture is in excellent shape, my bones are hard and durable and I enjoy rigorous physical activities. My alkalizing diet and overall healthful lifestyle have enabled my bones to fully remineralize. I have also learned the importance of maintaining a relaxed belly, a graceful curve in my lower spine for freeing up the flow of nerve energy to the abdominal organs, and breathing deeply and fully. With this plus my other lifestyle changes, my bowels are functioning perfectly with no trace of the past illness.

The wonderful thing about living a healthful lifestyle is that the pain of past memories has faded away in the glow of my new health!

The Fruits of Life

In 1987 I moved to northern California to be where organically grown produce is abundant, and where I would further pursue environmental engineering. Near San Francisco I met the prolific natural health and fitness writer Morris Krok, who has furthered my education on fruitarian diet and the value of yoga practices for keeping the body fit. Eight years into my rejuvenation I began to feel dynamically healthy and naturally euphoric.

In 1992 I left engineering to begin a career in health education and consulting. In 1993 I received a Nutrition Educator certification from the Institute for Educational Therapy (subsequently renamed Bauman College). I have since taught nutrition and self-healing education classes, worked as a health consultant, begun publishing *Living Nutrition* magazine, co-authored *Your Natural Diet: Alive Raw Foods,* and authored *Self Healing Colitis & Crohn's* and *The Art of Rejuvenation.* In 2006 I received a Ph.D./Hygienic Doctorate in Health and Natural Healing from the

University of Natural health. *Self Healing Colitis & Crohn's* served as my thesis.

Everyday I marvel at how I went from chronic fatigue, illness and misery to becoming a leader in the Natural Hygiene movement. For all of my teachers', friends' and family's support I am eternally grateful. Now, at age 51, I feel youthful and full of life. This I attribute to my raw fruit-based diet, daily exercise, positive thinking and passion for life. Obtaining an accurate educational foundation in nutrition and health was the key to my healing success. Regular vigorous exercise was essential in my rebuilding, and it continues to be important in maintaining my health. A favorite adage of mine, which I live by, is:

The body will not rebuild itself unless it is given
a reason to do so; only in response to exercise will
the body build a better body.

Afterword

The Crohn's and Colitis Foundation estimates that there are 1.5 million colitis and Crohn's disease sufferers in the United States. As always, the Foundation's positions are that there is no known cause of colitis and Crohn's disease, there is no known cure for colitis except for surgical removal of the colon, and diet is not a causative factor with these diseases. And millions worldwide are hearing that misinformation! In 1993 when I began to tell a Foundation spokeswoman about my story, she said, "Well good for you, but that doesn't work for everyone." After I pressed her, she said "I don't have time to listen to this," and she hung up her telephone. Today, the prevailing medical approach continues to be medicine, low-fiber, cooked-food diet with meat and last-resort surgery.

A small but growing number of others have found the Natural Hygiene solution to IBD as I did, including one M.D., Dr. Jack Goldstein, who wrote the now out-of-print book *Fasting Saved My Life!* Now, as a Hygienic Doctor and Director of the Colitis & Crohn's Health Recovery Center, I help people overcome IBD with consistent success. I have counseled over 2,000 people with crippling disease to new health and vitality, and this book has enjoyed remarkable acceptance worldwide including, in recent years, by some medical doctors. My colleague and dear friend, Dr. Zarin Azar, a gastroenterologist in Los Angeles, California, is the only medical doctor who has fully incorporated the program in my book into her practice.

It is my sincere wish that the natural healing alternative be embraced by the medical establishment and be revealed to the many IBD sufferers who deserve the same chance to recover as I had. While my recovery was unique, there are many pathways to health. However, it is certain that they are all grounded in biological truths...naturally!

6.4
I Live in Joy Now
(*David's Song of Life*)

I live in joy now
and the memories from the past
are distant and faded

I can only faintly remember:
the pain
the torture
the anguish
the agony
the aggravation
the confusion
the turmoil
the misery
the ugliness
the indignity
the disgust
the depression
the loneliness
the helplessness
the frustration
the despair
the hatred
the suffering
the emptiness
the lovelessness
the desperation
the fear
from the life that was a traumatic dying hell

That chapter in my life is long gone
I ended it on one glorious day a long time ago
I have reclaimed my health and my life

I love
I share
I sing
I live in joy now

6.5
TESTIMONIALS

"Since I changed to a natural diet as suggested by David, I am convinced that my body is totally free of colitis. I feel great and have more energy than I know!"
- Paul Nison, Brooklyn, New York (1997)

"Today I am in better health than ever! My healing has led me to become a natural health educator and author. I have referred many people to David and have learned that the ones who use this approach heal up every time."
– Paul Nison, Brooklyn, New York (2000)

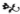

"For a couple of months I suffered with advanced ulcerative colitis after having colitis for 12 previous years. After consulting David, I studied his booklet, took myself off the prednisone and asacol I was taking, followed his dietary and healing advice, and it worked! I overcame my symptoms immediately and now, four months later, I feel I am totally healed of the illness. The doctors told me if I stopped the medications I would have a recurrence. I am sure they are wrong. I have no indigestion problems, I feel good about my new diet and about myself, and I credit David for inspiring me to achieve my new health."
– David T., Sun Lakes, Arizona (1998)

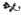

"I stuck to your program and it worked just as I always knew it would. I am not taking any of my old medications such as 6MP or Azulfadine any more!!! I did have a very tough 1-2 months back in September, but I toughed it out and sure enough I was okay. Believe me, I would have never thought that I would ever be off all medications again, had it not been for your books. I cannot thank you enough. If I ever go out to California again, I would like to meet with you to personally thank you. You have led me back to a health I thought I had lost for good. I am getting the "old me" back."
– Gregory C., Nanuet, New York (1998)

"I have Ileitis. I was diagnosed about 4 months ago. I feel like I want to die. I am on prednisone and azulfadine and I am getting worse. This is ruining my life. I've eaten terrible food my entire life and I am willing to try anything to be normal again. I hope this really works."

– Chad L., Germantown, Maryland (December, 1998)

"All is going well right now. I am back to work and living a normal life. I am not on any medicines. I am not fully keeping up with the diet, but I am changing slowly. I eat fruits and vegetables 500 times more than I ever did. I bought a juicer and I do that as much as I can. But I still eat 'bad' things more than I should. I am happy though and feel a lot better."

– Chad L., Germantown, Maryland (January, 1999)

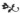

"The diet is going well! I'm really starting to feel great! A week ago over Christmas at home I really didn't feel like doing very much except lying around the house. Can you believe this morning I was out in 25 degree weather riding three miles on my mountain bike! And remember how I missed the ski trip to Aspen because I was feeling pretty poor and low on energy? Well, this weekend we're headed to Vermont to ski Stratton. I couldn't be happier—skiing is my TRUE passion! Things are only going to get better.

"I also wanted to let you know that on Monday I went in for a colonoscopy (at my request, not the doctor's) because I WANTED TO SEE what was going on inside MY body. I was tired of just getting the flexible sigmoidoscope done in the office and then having them explain to me what THEY saw. I needed to know and see for myself! Guess what? My colon is totally NORMAL—NO INFLAMMATION, NO ULCERATIONS AND NO CONSTRICTIONS. My doctor was completely thrilled. Now she said we just have to get my head clear from all the medicines. I'm down to 10 mg. on the prednisone and tomorrow I go to 7.5 mg. It won't be long until I'm totally off the stuff. I can't wait!"

– Krist D., Cos Cob, Connecticut (1999)

"I thought you might like to know that after I read *Self Healing Colitis & Crohn's,* I changed to a vegetarian, Natural Hygiene diet and immediately saw improvement! Previously, I was expelling gas, blood, and mucous, along with abnormal, frequent stools for months. Well, incredibly, these symptoms have almost disappeared. I went "off" the diet over the 4th of July weekend, and sure enough, the symptoms came back mildly, but I am amazed at how quickly I'm healing up."

– Donna B., Tarzana, California (1999)

"After having a biopsy in April 1999, I was told I had ulcerative colitis. This was no surprise as I'd had minor symptoms (bleeding) for a couple of years and my uncle and 2 cousins also have the illness. I was given suppositories which cleared it up, but over the summer I started feeling very fatigued and lethargic. I was getting almost constant gut pain (especially when I ate) and had no energy to do anything. I'd already got into juicing, which had started to give me more energy. After studying *Self Healing Colitis & Crohn's,* I realized that it wasn't just juicing that would make me better—I basically needed to embrace the whole package. I have gradually done this and can honestly say I feel fantastic for it. I found David's information on food and eating particularly useful and as soon as I applied the techniques, any gastric distress after meals completely stopped. It's as simple as that.

"Rather than telling you that you've got a terrible illness and trying to show you how to live with it, David's approach looks at the causes of colitis and Crohn's, and shows you how to eliminate them. There's therefore no breeding ground for the disease to occur. I would recommend *Self Healing Colitis & Crohn's* to anyone and think the medical profession should be ashamed of itself for not adopting it."

– Nick Ledger, York, England, <nickledger@ukjuicers.com> (1999)

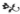

"I already have your book *Self Healing Colitis & Crohn's.* You have helped me to regain my health and my life! I can't thank you enough! I'm buying this one for a young friend who is struggling with colitis. Thanks again!"

– Dave F., Nashville, Tennessee (2000)

"I wanted to let you know how I am doing. We spoke last Tuesday night and I was feeling terrible. The next day, I purchased a juicer and started your program. With each day, I am getting better. In fact, yesterday (Sunday) I was as normal as I have been for almost a year."

– Tina H., Dayton, Ohio (2000)

"I feel that I am healed after seven weeks into the changed diet that you helped me with. Here is where I am at: At six weeks, there was no blood, and somewhat normal bm's. The urgency to go to the bathroom was there, but milder than before. Now at seven weeks, I feel I have more control over my bowels and only the slightest urgency. My bm's are blood free. Well, I am feeling so much better. I have no pain or bloating and I am elated!"

– Tina H., Dayton, Ohio (2000)

"I am in week eight, and I am doing great! I really feel healed, and shared the info with my internet message board people, with some sarcastic feedback from a couple, very negative, but for the most part, people are really intrigued. I pray that they get in touch with you. The negative ones were the ones saying that their quality of life was so bad, that giving up their favorite foods would essentially mess up their day. They cannot believe that changing their diet would really help. I feel disappointment for them, and hope that they will change their minds. Thank you so much for everything."

– Tina H., Dayton, Ohio (2000)

"Today I was thinking about the month of April as I watched my kids playing outside during a very beautiful and perfect spring day in Ohio. I then remembered that it was one year ago this month that I contacted you. I suddenly went back to how sick and miserable I felt, trying to live normally and looking for any available restroom. Today, I am still well. If you remember, it took me about eight weeks to fully recover. I remember by the first or second week of June I really felt normal again, and confident to admit to it, too. Thank you Dave. I am still teaching aerobics and lifting weights. I no longer fear going shopping or long trips. I followed your plan, and I try to live like a vegetarian with the exception of a little chicken every so often...that is it. I still think of all of your advice and I wanted to let you know that I feel great!"

– Tina H., Dayton, Ohio (2001)

"It is April, and two years of living in freedom and loving the fact that I rarely ever think of how sick I had been back in April of 2000. If you remember, you helped me and I will never forget it. Every April I start to think about it, and it is especially on my mind this time because a friend has the symptoms and is going through a hard time with a divorce that has caused her a great deal of stress, thus causing the colitis and blood. She will be in touch with you. I just wanted to take this time to share my thanksgiving of good health with you. However, I am worried for my friend. She is beautiful and intelligent and I am sure she will get in touch. Thanks for all you did for me. God Bless You!

– Tina H., Dayton, Ohio (2002)

※

"Okay Dave, this is something. Today for the first time in nearly three months I've started to have formed stools with very little blood—this after only a day and a half on your diet plan! To say I'm encouraged by this is an understatement. To say I'm a little skeptical about the long term results because of the nature of this disease would be an honest observation. But I'm the eternal optimist so I'm going to continue doing as you directed and see what happens, expecting continued improvement in my colon and overall health. Thank you so much for sharing what you have learned."

– John O., Tulsa, Oklahoma (2000)

"I'm John, from Tulsa, who left a couple of testimonials on your website back in 2000 about the success I experienced after our phone consultation and following your general recommendations for my recently diagnosed, chronic UC condition.

"I'm happy to report I'm still UC symptom-free! In fact, a person just contacted me yesterday asking me questions about how I found success and I pointed them to your website — just as I've done before when people ask the same.

"So, I just wanted to say THANK YOU once again and that your advice certainly isn't a quick-fix treatment or something that doesn't last. I'm a walking, breathing testimony to that!"

– John O., Tulsa, Oklahoma (2007)

"The last time we spoke you had called me on the phone and I had just come out of the hospital, back in November. It's been one heck of a ride since then. I won't explain every detail here, but I am doing fantastically now. My mental and physical energies are higher than they were before the colitis started, and my emotions have become more stable as I have begun to take an observational attitude towards all three aspects of my personality. Now the great news: I am currently on the verge of attaining super-health. The wisdom and strength that I have gained and received from traversing this path are enormous. The difference between "hearing about," "reading about," "intelligently being aware of" and really KNOWING on a cellular level what the Truth is about is awesome. My overall gratitude and appreciation for the loving work that you and others have done only increases."

– Jason Hebert, Marshfield, Massachusetts (2000)

"Dave, these are the best bowel movements I've every had after a lifetime of constipation with years of Crohn's. It's effortless—like a marvel. I've been on your diet for two weeks and it's not as hard as I thought it would be. I'm on no medications and feel great. I can't thank you enough. After searching and trying alternative therapies for years, your help has been invaluable."

– Lois C., Cherry Hill, New Jersey (2000)

"I had to let you know that the information you sent me two weeks ago, *Self Healing Colitis & Crohn's,* has been nothing short of lifesaving and inspirational! I'm just presently healing from a severe case of colitis. I've been on all the drugs, asacol, prednisone, sulfa, and all they did was cause more problems. This has been the most devastating thing that has ever happened to me, I thought I would certainly die from it. I found the information you sent me to be the most valuable and detailed to date. I re-read the material every day to give me hope and guidance and have incorporated many of your ideas into my diet. So, thanks again for all the wonderful information, positive outlook and support. I know I wouldn't be this far along without your advice!"

   – Gary A., Alta Loma, California (2000)

"It was very upsetting to be told that our twelve-year old son had an 'incurable' disease, but *Self Healing Colitis & Crohn's* offered us a ray of hope. Straight after the colonoscopy we started the natural diet. After four days Jacob called us to the loo in great excitement to see formed stools for the first time since his problems began two months ago! After a week of further celebration, no blood! Today the gastroenterologist reduced me to tears. She became really angry when I told her about the diet and said that in her 35 years of experience none of her patients had ever been "cured" by diet and those who had tried had suffered more in the long run. It's doubly difficult to defy the medical profession as a parent because you are accused of being irresponsible to your child's detriment. How I hope we can prove them wrong!"

   – Deborah D., Caesaria, Israel (2001)

"We would never be able to thank you enough! It is now six months and Jacob has continued to be entirely healthy and symptom-free from Crohn's. It is amazing how he has turned his diet around completely and found that he really enjoys healthful food and does not crave animal products. Jacob was a sworn avocado hater, but you suggested he mash avocado into potato which he did and liked, and gradually avocado became one of his favorite foods. He has even invented his own pasta sauce with avocado and fresh tomatoes, and it is delicious! I have written to my doctor and hospital telling them of our success. I hope they take notice. Thank you so much; your advice was a lifeline and your telephone consultations helped us so much at the beginning. You saved Jacob, now age 13, from a life of medication and operations and you are brilliant! If you ever decide to visit this country again you must come and visit us."

   – Deborah D., Caesaria, Israel (2001)

"We just wanted to drop you a note to thank you for your work. Our daughter Caroline, age 13, is completely off all drugs and has not had a flare-up in six months. Your research and lifetime commitment have allowed our daughter to

have a normal adolescence free of drugs. Thank God for people like you who dare to question the medical establishment. Keep up the good work."
– Tony and Laura F., Lexington, Kentucky (2001)

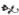

"Thank you for returning my call. I must say I was very impressed that you called. I received your book, and what an eye opener it has been for me. I've stopped eating all meat products and I'm amazed that I don't even have a craving for them. My diet consists primarily of vegetables and fruits. I wanted to let you know that I haven't had one bout of diarrhea in over a week. All I can say is, "Yippee, Hooray" and all that good stuff! I mean this sincerely, because I have experienced diarrhea almost every day for a year. My husband has noticed that I have more energy, and even my skin tone has improved. All of this in just one week. I also realize that I still have work to do in order to continue the healing process, but in just one week I am feeling much better. Thank you for sharing your wisdom and outstanding knowledge so that others might experience optimum health and happiness. Your book should be on every Best Sellers list."
– Cindy G., Las Vegas, Nevada (2001)

"The diet you advocate afforded me wonderful improvement. My bowel and arthritic episodes were brought down to a sustainable pain level after 2 to 3 weeks following a flare-up. I wanted to pass on some information should you encounter someone with polyarthritis in conjunction with Crohn's. I searched all the arthritis and allergy web sites for vegetable foods that trigger arthritic episodes. I subsequently removed corn (acid forming), cabbage, peas (metabolic waste produced by digestion of cabbage and peas is hippuric acid which obviously my liver cannot detoxify) and the nightshade family (which contain a toxin called solanine which my liver cannot handle) from my diet. I have been juicing cabbage daily and eating peas, tomatoes, sweet peppers and potatoes on a daily basis as well. I also removed all acid forming protein sources from my diet: nuts, seeds, coconut and olives. After 4 days the pain finally released its grip on my body. I feel human again."
– Kim-Mia M., Calgary, Alberta, Canada (2001)

"I began the new health program with hopes that this would cure my 3-year Crohn's illness and fistulas, or at least make my life a lot better. I noticed a major difference on Day 3, when my cramps, mouth ulcers and pimples began disappearing and my stools became smaller and very easy to pass. Having a bowel movement had become pleasurable at last! In just 3 days the blood discharge had reduced from a great amount to a trickle, and most of the pain had subsided. My energy level became good as the program apparently started to work. The bleeding further diminished within a week, then for the next 7 days I had no symptoms at all: no bleeding, cramping and no large stools."

– Ryan P., Sidney, Australia (2001)

" I can't thank you enough Dave for all that you have done for me. You have shown me the simple truth. The world is truly blessed to have you as a teacher of Natural Hygiene. Thanks so much Dave! Take care mate!"

– Ryan P., Sidney, Australia (2007)

❧

"I have to thank you so much for changing my life. I went to see my consultant and he said there is a big change within three weeks. I am healing up and am in week 7 of my diet. How can I thank you again?!!"

– Pam M., London, England (2001)

❧

"I am delighted to be writing to you with my great news. Since I spoke to you a few months ago and since I have started my new diet, my whole life has changed. I have given up meat completely; however, I did have one slice of turkey on Christmas day, but I didn't feel the better for it. It felt really heavy in my tummy. Imagine how I would have felt if I had eaten a lot of it! So I will not be tempted next year. I have had no pain at all really, I have gone back to my original clothes size and I have a flat tummy! My body looks great and I feel great!!

"I want to thank you and whatever Angels helped you when you were sick for finding this diet and sharing it with the world. Lots of things have happened to me and life at the moment is terrific. Thank you so much."

– Sinead O., Dublin, Ireland (2001)

❧

"I contacted you from a hospital in Orange County in October and November, 2000. I was suffering from acute ulcerative colitis. I was down from my ideal weight of 175 pounds to 130 pounds. The doctors were strongly advising me to have my colon surgically removed. I thought that was a little drastic so I asked my sisters, Cathy and Dian, to check on wholistic approaches to the disease and they put me in touch with you.

"As a result of your advice and a lot of independent reading and study of my own, I went on an all-vegetable juice and fruit smoothie diet for about 2 months. Then I gradually started adding back solid foods starting with soft non-acidic fruits. I also gradually weaned myself from all of the drugs the doctors had me on. You were absolutely right in that I did not really start recovering until I stopped taking all the drugs. By January of 2001 I was feeling much better and I was well on my way to recovery.

"Now, a year later, I am back to my original 175 pounds and I am partaking in all the activities that I love like snow skiing, bicycling, hiking, etc. From your advice and the assistance of my sisters, I survived my stay in the hospital and I am pretty much back to normal now. The only real difference in my life is that I am now a vegetarian, although not a perfectly strict one. I wanted to take this opportunity to thank you and encourage you to keep up the good work. By the way, if anyone ever requests to talk to one of the people you have helped with colitis, I will be glad to do so."

– David L., Los Angeles, California (2002)

"I just got my last blood test results and they are nearly back to normal. The specialist still says I am very lucky to be alive as he thought my bowel was about to perforate around last Christmas. I will never forget e-mailing you the day after Christmas absolutely distraught because the bleeding had become severe, pouring out of me. I was in severe pain, not able to sit up, and very weak. I am eternally grateful that I did not take the Prednisone and immediately went on your diet. When feeling fragile and scared it helped me tremendously that you were able to strongly support my decisions. I am now better and eating fruits and vegetables. I know I will have to be very careful about what I do eat. I am grateful for your book and thank you once again. I truly believe and know you have saved my life."

– Shona C., Auckland, New Zealand (2002)

"I want to say you are a huge inspiration in my life, and your books and web sites have been amazingly helpful. Your magazine *Living Nutrition* magazine is AMAZING, and I just recently purchased all the back issues. I could continue the praise, but I know you are busy. I am a 26-year-old medical doctor (graduated last year), and I had to quit my family practice residency because of Crohn's disease. I got no relief from anywhere except your methods. Thank You, you are truly a saint!!"

—Mike Aquilina, M.D., Easton, Maryland, (2002)

"I went to a nutritionist in Manchester who referred me to David Klein's web site, www.colitis-crohns.com. I purchased his book *Self Healing Colitis & Crohn's* and followed the diet as best I could. Within four days, I was jumping around for joy—I was finally back to normal: no cramps, diarrhea or blood. I felt the life flowing back into me. I just couldn't believe how good I felt—I wanted to go straight to David Klein's house and give him a huge hug!

"Since I started the diet in June, I have had absolutely no pains or signs that they would return. I still follow the diet, but have added a few things now and again to keep me happy! I am not on any drugs as I feel it is wrong to keep taking drugs for life. It really is a healthy and fulfilling diet and lifestyle, and it's not hard to follow and well worth it."

—David Remnant, Manchester, England, (2003)

"I've now been on the diet for six weeks and off my meds! I'm feeling wonderful! I've noticed some great improvement in my reflexes. After my motorcycle accident in July of 1993, my reflexes were awfully slow. However, after being on this diet for just six weeks, my reflexes are much improved. Also the ulcerative colitis is in total remission without meds! I'm able to take my golden retriever each day again for a run by my 3-wheel bike! He loves it! When I wasn't feeling well, he'd lay right beside me. I'm doing good and expect things to keep getting better. Thanks so much!"

– Paula P., Wenatchee, Washington (2005)

"I contacted you several weeks ago in regard to your counseling services and your book, which I have since ordered and read. After many years of intestinal distress, I have been symptom-free for nearly two weeks. I am strictly eating fruit mono meals and occasional freshly-juiced vegetables. I cannot thank you enough for the information I received from your website and book. At 21 years old, I never thought I would lead a normal life and experience the feeling of health and vitality that I have now enjoyed glimpses of. I am urging my entire family to follow this path, and they are also trying. (We have a long history of intestinal cancer.)

"I keep finding myself at your website again, whenever I am looking for relevant information. I am a University student in my fourth year. Health and nutrition have always been huge concerns for me, as well as passions. When I stumbled upon the Natural Hygiene Courses I was more than intrigued. I am very interested in the programs, and would appreciate as much information or guidance you could provide."

– Carina Honga, Vancouver, Canada (2005)

"I ordered your book and will be calling you in a week or so. I went to a Colitis and Crohn's Foundation of America support group this evening and ran into a woman on your diet. She was very happy and I was glad to see living proof that this program works."

– Verneta G., Los Angeles, California (2005)

"Your program has been a Godsend for me. I haven't taken any meds in years after being diagnosed with ulcerative colitis. As long as I stay on your program I continue to get better. I encourage anybody suffering with ulcerative colitis or Crohn's to try your program. It works! Thanks again for all your great work."

– Dan Halverson, Newton, Massachusetts (2005)

"Thank you again. One year later I still feel like a million bucks."

– S.A., Danbury Connecticut (2005)

"I completely healed myself from colitis on your diet program. Your work on nutrition has saved my life and I want to thank you from the bottom of my heart. I have now left behind a terrible life and started to live with laws of nature. Thank you so much!

"I was diagnosed with colitis in March, 2005. I actually was sick from October, 2004, but I did not see a gastroenterologist for a proper diagnosis until my condition became severe. In March, after a colonoscopy and biopsy of a colon tissue, the doctor confirmed moderate ulcerative colitis in rectal and sigmoid area. When he told me that I would have to live on medicine the rest of my life, an image of a handicapped and crippled life loomed over me and I cannot tell in words how depressed I was for many months, especially at my young age (24 years). I was making good progress in my career, but all my dreams came to a sudden halt. I cried at night back then.

"In my continuous search on the Internet for a colitis cure, I found a natural diet program book which gave some direction about improving the diet. However, it included blended peanuts and other nuts and rough fiber which caused even more severe bleeding. In January, 2006 I read your book and went on an all-juice diet for almost 40 days while taking a thorough rest (mostly in bed) and I healed completely.

"But right after my healing, my cravings were tremendous for eating my old favorite foods, so I bought a fancy raw food recipe book. I made so many recipes for the next three months and ate so much that I undermined the healing. Most of the entrées included a large amount of nuts and seeds. Then my friend invited me to her graduation party at an Italian restaurant where I ate lot of bad food. On that day I began to see the colitis symptoms again.

"At that point I stopped eating anything bad and restarted the juice diet and reread your book over and over. I began to understand the power of fruits and the damage that cooked protein will cause. In two months I became completely symptom-free.

"Now, I eat very simply. I have eaten 390 bananas since June. I am going to eat three bananas for lunch for the rest of my life.

"Thank you so much. I'm enjoying a wonderful life now. Colitis troubled me so much, but it taught me a big lesson I needed to learn. I would like to thank you in person some time."

– Manish Kumar Jain, Department of Chemical Engineering, University of Houston, Houston, Texas (2006)

"I send people to your website. I hope they have the discipline and wisdom to follow through. I'm feeling great with no problems at all since 2000 after following your program. Colitis was a godsend to get me into a new way of life. And you were there at the time I needed you and I will always be grateful. The Vegan Healing Diet (along with playing blues guitar) is the best way I know of for feeling great! Here's a poem I wrote:"

Ode to David

I once had colitis
so the doctor gave me pills
he said: "son, now you take these
for all your pains and ills"

So I took those little red things.
they didn't do a lot
except make me even sicker
and tied my stomach in a knot!

I said: "Doc you must be kidding—
surely there's a cure"
he said: "no, son, I'm truly sorry"
then he gave me more!

Then I found this guy named David Klein
I heard what he had to say
and threw away those little red pills
and have been a new man since that day!

– Ralph Acerno, River Edge, New Jersey (2006)

"I bought *Self Healing Colitis & Crohn's* last November and found it to be what I was looking for over the last 12 years. It basically kept me away from a colostomy.

"For the past 12 years, I have gone through very difficult times with ulcerative colitis and was under a lot of pressure from my GI doctor and surgeon to have a colostomy. Thank God I was able to resist.

"After applying the healing plan in the book I am much better and currently leading almost a normal life.

"I appreciate your help Dave—you have shown me how to deal with this monstrous disease."

– Abu M., Saudi Arabia (2006)

"I was at the point of total desperation when I made one last ditch effort to find an alternative cure. If not for your guidance, I would have gone back to the doctor and agreed to take Remicade as the last resort. But I ran across your book and went on the program. After three weeks I am doing so much better. I had to gradually make the adjustments but they are long-term and I feel 80% better. I will be a true advocate of the program and a lifelong follower. I am sure I am headed for full recovery of my Crohn's. I have suffered horribly with this condition and the relief now is wonderful. I want to thank you. I owe you so much."

– Becky L., Alton, Missouri (2006)

"I am the bodybuilder formerly with ulcerative colitis who spoke to you five weeks ago. I have followed the diet you recommended since then. I was already on the diet outlined in your book for about two weeks prior to our talking. Your consultation helped me fine tune my eating for better results. The diet has helped me get progressively better and, as of the last five days, I have been absolutely symptom-free! It's fortunate that I caught this problem early, lost only 12 pounds

while detoxing and never had to use steroids. I love my new energy levels! And that's after only seven to eight weeks. I imagine how I'm going to feel a year with this new eating lifestyle...because I'm never going back to the SAD diet again!"
– John C., Phoenix, Arizona (2007)

⁂

"I just completed four of the eight weeks I needed to make up for lost time at med school. It was pretty demanding, but I remained loyal to the diet and made it through just fine. I have this week off to rejuvenate, before I have to go back for the remaining four weeks. You've done no less than give me my life back and I can't thank you enough for that.

"I've come to learn that my story is not much different from that of other IBD sufferers. I was living a happy and healthy life when one day, for no apparent reason, I suddenly began to experience abdominal cramps and loose stools. Over time, this progressed to debilitating abdominal pain and 20-plus bloody and mucoid bowel movements each day.

"As I am training to be a medical doctor, I naturally turned to traditional medicine for answers. Definitive answers were not what I got. Nonetheless, traditional medicine was all I knew. So, despite my obvious gaps in knowledge on this matter, I took a leap of faith and followed the directions given to me. I tried just about every anti-inflammatory, anti-spasmodic, and over-the-counter analgesic available. I went through numerous courses of steroids and even an immunosuppressant. For about a year I let the doctors adjust and readjust medication dosages in the hope that they would eventually find the key and would be able to protect me from having a colectomy.

"During this year, life as I knew it was over. I had to take leave from school, lost about 60 pounds, spent 10 days in the hospital, experienced indescribable abdominal pain, became housebound due to the frequency of bowel movements, took 20 or more pills a day, incurred numerous side effects from these various medications, and spent thousands of dollars on treatments that did not help.

"My observations led me to believe that the treatments I was given were actually worsening my condition. But what could I do? After all, I had to follow the advice of my experienced doctors, right? Wrong. One day, I finally realized that if all these medications weren't helping, then how could I justify the side effects and expense? The doctors strongly advised me to continue the treatment, but I was slowly and painfully dying at the age of 27, and nothing that they were doing for me was of any help. In the case of IBD, traditional medicine did not have an answer for me and I needed to look elsewhere.

"Everything changed for me when I MIRACULOUSLY found your *Self Healing Colitis & Crohn's* book online. I likely would have dismissed your theories as nonsense if I had come across them during the first month of the illness. But I was now in month 11 and was meeting with a surgeon to discuss a colectomy. So, I read your book and for the first time felt like someone else understood my predicament. The things you said were in direct agreement with my own experiences and observations. For the first time in a long time, I was filled with hope and felt as if this illness might be manageable.

"I am now at month 15 and have been free of medications and doctor visits. I've spoken to you numerous times over the telephone and through e-mail. You have done nothing less than nurse me back to health and given me my life back. How do you repay someone for that?

"Many of the doctors I work with are quite interested in hearing my story. They are astonished that detox and diet have played such a crucial role in my healing. Such a concept remains foreign to allopathic physicians. A few of those doctors tell me that they have heard similar stories from some of their own patients but, in the end, they have no training or understanding of nutrition and natural healing and can do little more than simply listen to my story."

– S.G., Florida (2007)

"It will be three years in May since I first contacted you. I was having upsetting digestive problems and had a colonoscopy that showed the beginnings of colitis and Crohn's disease. I purchased your book, we had a long consultation, and I switched to vegetarianism. Although I have somewhat modified the program over the years, not a day goes by that I don't have at least eight to ten fresh fruits plus veggies. I have canceled all meat, fish and poultry from my diet.

"I recently had my annual physical examination with my doctor. He wanted me to have a colonoscopy. I hadn't had one in three years and was curious to see what it would show. Thank G-d, it was excellent! Now I am 58 years old, and no signs of any Crohn's disease, colitis, diverticulitis or polyps!

"This diet has transformed my whole life. Your wisdom that you share with others makes you a true miracle worker. Thank you so much and G-d bless you for your teachings and the wonderful work you do to help others."

– Jacqueline K., Los Angeles, California (2007)

"My son Byron (who in 2006 at age 17 was diagnosed with Crohn's) recently confided in me that one year ago he wanted to commit suicide. At that time he was confined to bed with painful fissures, anal tears, mouth ulcers, stomach cramps, diarrhea, bowel incontinence, hot and cold sweats and a host of other miserable complaints. He had endured months of illness and hospitalization and, despite drug treatments, he was not improving.

"Then your Self Healing Colitis & Crohn's book arrived. He began the diet immediately and within three days the fissure pain was gone and he was up and moving around.

"We have since proved every single word of your book to be true. Byron's recovery went exactly as you described it would. He followed the steps carefully, reducing the drugs.

"We know your work has saved Byron from a life of hell. Today, one year after receiving your book, he is entirely drug-and-symptom-free. His weight has increased from 45 kg to 62 kg. He is an active young man who looks and feels great. I am also very happy to report that he now has a vegan girlfriend.

"Byron lives by the Vegan Post-healing Diet and finds it easy to stick with. We spend far less time on food preparation than we did before, and we now spend absolutely no money on drugs, supplements or medical consultations.

"When the doctor recently labeled Byron's excellent condition 'clinical remission,' we confidently told him this will continue for about another 75 years!

"Byron and I believe you have provided him with the 'cure.' Over the six months prior to receiving your book, his medical treatments cost approximately AUS$15,000. Your regimen cost us only the price of the book and one in-person consultation fee when I was fortuitously able to meet with you in California last year.

"We thank you for so much. Please add Byron's story to your list of testimonials. I am happy to have my e-mail address posted on your website for those who read your "Are You Skeptical" section, and I will be pleased to share our story."

–Julie Smith, Australia, <jsm58010@bigpond.net.au> (2008)

"I wanted to let you know how well things are going for me. I had consulted with you a few times this past winter. I'm not sure exactly what has happened within my body over these months, but it's been miraculous and I credit you and your writing for much of it!

"For months I had struggled to implement the healing diet. I slowly switched to an all-organic diet and made some progress, but I was still eating grains and a lot of poor food combinations. A few weeks after I entirely cut out grains, I noticed, incredibly, that I was no longer craving them—or anything unhealthy—anymore! My cravings virtually disappeared and my colitis symptoms started to subside as well.

"About two months ago when I was still not feeling completely well and was experiencing digestive symptoms, I lost my appetite and simply stopped eating. I fasted for about five days on just water and my energy, vitally and mental clarity absolutely soared! I had fasted many times before but had never experienced this effect. What's even more interesting is that when I did finally decide to eat again, I only wanted one thing: raw fruit!

"Of all the benefits I've received, the lack of food cravings astounds me most. I have literally forgotten what it even feels like to want and crave unhealthy food!

"Thank you for all your writings and hard work. You led me from a very dark place into the light."

–Adam F., Connecticut (2008)

"Thank you so much for your excellent book. I'm going to call it my Bible! It's been two months since I last spoke with you and I want to let you know the diet has helped tremendously. I had a colonoscopy last month and I cannot believe the pictures of the lower colon—it healed beautifully!

"I have been recommending your book to lots of people and doctors as well."

–Clarey G., California (2008)

"I am writing to thank you and express the joy that your book has brought back into my life. I had suffered from ulcerative colitis since 1996 with several hospital stints and dark periods of illness. When I came across your book on the Internet 18 months ago I implemented the plan partially and noticed a marked improvement in my overall health. Three months ago I decided to fully comply with the plan and now I enjoy full health and happiness.

"I find the subject of raw food nutrition to be so fascinating that I am considering changing my career into that field. Western medicine needs to wake up to these fundamental truths."

–Allan C., Ireland (2008)

"I have good news to report: over the past two and one-half weeks I have been feeling much better with one regular bowel movement per day and no bad digestive symptoms. The horrible arthritic joint pain is gone and the horrible skin inflammation is almost gone. Thank you so much for your help! The natural diet plan along with my fervent prayers have truly restored my health and life in ten weeks!"

–Margaret W., Ohio (2009)

6.6
CONCLUSION

C&C are degenerative illnesses which are caused by chronic stress from any of the following sources: diet, lifestyle, the mind, emotions, society, culture and environment. The stressors result in physiological enervation and toxification of the human organism, leading to the heightened, distressful elimination and inflammation responses which are properly referred to as "detoxification dis-ease."

In virtually every case, health is restorable and the diseases will not return if the healthful living practices taught herein are correctly practiced. In order to restore health, persons with C&C should be cared for wholistically—the causes of disease must be discontinued, healthful practices must be implemented and the detoxification process must be allowed to proceed to completion. The body will be guided by its innate intelligence and naturally heal itself when all the factors of health are in place. In order for complete healing, there must be an accurate understanding of the disease process, our biological needs and the overall health picture. Wholistic health guidance should be enlisted and self-education taken up.

All of the principles and assertions espoused herein are based on physiological fact and empirical experience—not on theories. The Natural Hygiene self-healing plan with the Vegan Healing Diet work because they are based on the immutable laws governing human biology and physiology. When we discontinue unhealthful practices and provide the requisites of health, eating our natural biological diet, the body will only improve itself, reversing disease and creating new health.

Natural self-healing has been around for a long time, dating back to biblical times. The Natural Hygiene movement began in the early 1800s and has continued to this day. Natural healing is actually nature's way. The body is programmed to self-heal. Many people who have followed the natural healing route for every known disease condition and have gone on to higher levels of health than ever before. To prove this true, each person must do the work and experience it for himself or herself. Healing and excellent health will come to fruition if one uses his or her higher intelligence and passionately embraces healthful living as a way of life.

The elements of an effective plan for overcoming C&C will vary from case to case. Generally speaking, the basics are: 1. Natural Hygiene education; 2. a natural, whole foods vegan diet (preferably organic) with juicing; 3. extra sleep and complete rest (sabbatical from work or school); 4. proper exercise; 5. health counseling; 6. peer support; and 7. medical cooperation. And each person must focus on giving him-herself nurturing love, living in harmony with nature and seeking out others who will support that goal wholeheartedly.

I wrote these words almost 26 years after I began my healing—my lasting healing—with guidance from my coaches and saviors Drs. Laurence Galant and T. C. Fry. Dr. Fry has passed on, yet I often give silent thanks to this lionhearted man for putting out and supporting me with the Natural Hygiene program information I direly needed. Dr. Galant is still my dear friend; we regularly speak on the phone and I occasionally visit him and express my gratitude and share my joy. You too can have 25 years of health freedom and happiness—simply dedicate yourself to healthful living and get the help you need. Healthful abundance awaits you. It's up to you—it only gets easier and easier and more and more joyful—naturally! Imagine it, visualize it, believe in your magnificent self-healing power, your God-given right to be healthy and your natural place in this world, and say: "I can do it!" You can! Celebrate your uniqueness, your sensitivity, your wisdom, your determination, love your self-healing body and keep on the healthful living path for life!

Note: If you are considering making any changes in your dietary and healing regime, please re-read Section 1.3, Advisory and the entire contents of this book many times and do not proceed unless you have a solid understanding of the safe and proper protocol to follow. Improper, hurried, misguided implementation of the healing diet plan espoused herein can be harmful. Dr. Klein and his qualified associates are available to properly assist clients.

7
APPENDICES

A
NUTRITION AND HEALTH GUIDANCE BY DR. DAVID KLEIN

I offer nutrition and health education, personalized diet and healing plans, guidance and ongoing support. Everyone who follows my guidance, with a 100% commitment to becoming healthy, heals up and rejuvenates. I'd like to emphasize that because everyone is at a different level of illness and has different needs, diet and healing plans must be personalized—there is no one standard dietary and healing formula; everyone needs special attention. Via consultation with the client, I am able to formulate proper personalized plans. I offer consultations by phone or in my office. I welcome your inquiry about how my educational and healing guidance services can help you. You may request my Health Questionnaire by e-mailing dave@colitis-crohns.com.

I am happy to help you overcome illness and create everlasting wellness!

David Klein, Ph.D., Director
Colitis & Crohn's Health Recovery Center
Phone: (707) 829-0462 * (877) 740-6082
Fax: (240) 414-5341
Mail: Post Box 256, Sebastopol, CA 95473 USA
E-mail: dave@colitis-crohns.com
Colitis & Crohn's Health Recovery Center web site:
www.colitis-crohns.com

Note: If this book is helping you to overcome illness and improve the quality of your life, please let me know. I am grateful for any and all feedback. Healing testimonial stories are welcomed.

B

HEALTH QUESTIONNAIRE

Colitis & Crohn's Health Recovery Center

Notes:

1. You may request a copy of this Health Questionnaire by e-mailing dave@ colitis-crohns.com, or you may fax this to Dr. Klein at (240) 414-5341. A digital copy may be downloaded from www.colitis-crohns.com/counseling.html.

2. A signed copy of the consultant-client agreement is required— see the end of this appendix.

3. A signed copy of the agreement may be mailed to: Colitis & Crohn's Health Recovery Center, P.O. Box 256, Sebastopol, CA 95473.

4. It is the client's responsibility to contact Dr. Klein and set up the consultations. The client makes the phone calls.

5. Prepayment by check or payment by credit card on the day when services are rendered is required. Contact Dr. Klein for his billing rate. Phone: (707) 829-0462 or (877) 740-6082.

E-mail: dave@colitis-crohns.com.

Consultation times: Monday through Thursday, 10:00 AM – 3:00 PM Pacific Standard Time.

Name:

Date:

Mail address:

Phone number:

E-mail address:

Where did you find my health education services?

Consultation payment method:
Credit card number and expiration date:

Age: Height: Weight:

Medical diagnosis:

Describe recent weight loss or gain:

Occupation:

Are you now working or in school?
How many hours per day?
Are you or your family dependent on your income?
Are you under any financial stress?
Are you on disability or considering it?
Are you on sabbatical or planning to take one?
Are you under any family stress?

Will your family support you in making diet and lifestyle changes?

Describe your recent and current health problem(s) and symptoms:

Describe your digestion (gas/stomach distress/etc.) and when problems occur:

Describe your bowel movement form, difficulties and frequency (e.g., diarrhea/stools/straining/bleeding/mucous/pains):

Do you have inflammation now?

Do you have a fever now, or have you had a fever recently?

How long have you been ill with a colon or intestinal problem?

Are you now under medical care?
Please describe:

Are you aware of, or being treated for, any nutritional deficiencies?

Have you had any blood chemistry tests? (Please attach copies).

Describe past health problems:

Describe past and present medications, alcohol, tobacco and recreational drug use:

Describe your energy levels during the day and evening:

How many hours of sleep do you get?

Do you take rests and naps during the day?

What is your health goal?

Have you thoroughly read and studied *Self Healing Colitis & Crohn's* (at least 5 times is recommended)?

Please list questions you have about *Self Healing Colitis & Crohn's*:

What are your favorite foods?

What foods do you normally or sometimes crave?

Describe your eating habits, how much you eat, and any recent trends in you diet:

What approximate percentage of your entire diet did the following foods make up before making any diet changes, if you made any changes when did you do so, and what approximate percent of your entire diet do these foods make up now:

Meat:
Dairy:
Cereals/pastas/bread/grains/pastries:
Fresh/raw fruit:
Cooked vegetables & potatoes:
Fresh/raw vegetables:
Raw nuts and seeds:
Beans/legumes:
Snacks (e.g., crackers, cookies, chocolate, ice-cream, candies, etc.):
Carbonated soft drinks:
Coffee:
Tea:

What is the approximate percentage of your diet that is raw/uncooked food?

Do you use table salt?

Do you use spices or seasonings?

Do you use bottled salad dressings or mayonnaise?

Please list any supplements/vitamins/nutrition powders you take.

If you eat meat, do you believe you can or cannot give it up?

Do you have any food allergies?
Please describe:

What kind of water do you drink, and how much?

Do you ever drink chlorinated city water?

Is your household water chlorinated, and if so, do you have a shower filter?

Do you have a juicer?
Do you have a steamer?

How is your appetite?
Do you wake up hungry?

Are you able to exercise?
Please describe what kinds and how much:

What are your favorite leisure time activities/hobbies?

Do you have a spiritual practice, such as meditation, prayer, etc.?

Please describe any parts of your body and life that you do not like:

What is your attitude toward your colon and bowel function?

Please describe any fears, shame and worries you have and how much you believe they are affecting your health and happiness:

Please describe any other kind of health support or therapy you are now receiving:

How quickly do you want to go with your diet and healthful lifestyle transition?

What would you like to learn more about?

Please attach additional information, such as diet and health diaries and lab reports.

Colitis & Crohn's Health Recovery Center

HEALTH DIARY FOR (NAME):

1. Date

2. Weight in lbs.

3. How I felt today

4. Energy level

5. Symptoms

6. Main concerns/struggles

7. Questions I have

8. Healing signs

9a. No. of BMs
9b. Diarrhea?
9c. Blood?
9d. Mucous?

10a. No. of hours of sleep
10b. No. of hours of rest
10c. No. of hours of work/chores
10d. No. of hours of exercise
10e. Type of exercise

11. Total water intake in quarts or 8 oz. glasses

12. Morning foods/drinks and quantity

13. Midday foods/drinks and quantity

14. Afternoon foods/drinks and quantity

15. Evening foods/drinks and quantity

16. Seasonings

17. Supplements

18. Medications and dosage

19. Therapies

20. Medical advice received today

21. Natural Hygiene literature I read today

22. Tests and health medical exams I am planning

23. Healing and lifestyle plans I am making

24. My affirmation of the day

25a. Need to set up a consultation with Dr. Klein?
25b. When?

26. Other info

Colitis & Crohn's Health Recovery Center

Client Statements of Understanding and Agreement

(Required)

I _____ (Client) agree to consult Dr. David Klein (Consultant) of Colitis & Crohn's Health Recovery Center for self-healing, health education and counseling services at the following pay rate:

_____.

The Client understands that:

* The Consultant is not a medical doctor nor a physician.

* The Consultant does not diagnose, treat or advise in medical areas.

* The Consultant is a Hygienic Doctor with a degree in Natural Health and Healing from the University of Natural Health, concentrating on educating and guiding people with inflammatory bowel disease to recover their health via implementing healthful living practices.

* The Consultant is also a Nutrition Educator, educated, trained and legally certified by the state of California through Bauman College to counsel people in matters of nutrition and health.

* The Consultant welcomes working in concert with medical doctors and registered nurses of the Client's choice.

* The Consultant's ability to provide effective healing counseling services is dependent upon the completeness and depth of information provided by the Client and his/her medical doctor.

* The Consultant requires that the Client promptly notify the Consultant of any great concern related to healing or illness symptoms, pains, or difficulties; if the Client deviates from the Consultant's guidance; if the Client is confused; and if the Client undergoes any kind of new, increased or decreased medical or non-medical treatment.

* The Consultant's goal is to help the Client self-heal his/her illness condition and become healthier in a manner which is safe and comfortable.

* The best healing results are realized via a complete rest of a duration which is dictated by the Client's physiological needs.

* The Consultant can only work with the Client if his/her family and advising medical doctor support the approach advised by the Consultant.

* The Consultant can only work with the Client if his/her goal is to make a safe, medically-approved transition off all drug therapies for inflammatory bowel disease as well as other non-recommended "healing remedies."

* There is some risk in this and any detoxification program. In all cases of inflammatory bowel disease, the body is already in an accelerated detoxification mode due to an overload of disease-causing toxic matter in the body. In the process of completely eliminating this toxic matter under the Consultant's natural detoxification plan, increased symptoms are temporarily experienced by a small percentage of Clients. Also, detoxification causes every client to experience temporary weight loss as toxic matter is eliminated. The Consultant strives to avoid detoxification problems. If detoxification symptoms including weight loss do begin to become extreme, the Consultant will recommend modifications of the Client's diet and self-healing program, aiming to slow down the detoxification process to a safe, more comfortable pace. If at any time during the self-healing program detoxification concerns cannot be quickly resolved, it is the Client's responsibility to obtain medical help as needed.

* The Consultant requires that Client take full responsibility for his/her decisions and actions and communicate with the Consultant in a courteous, respectful manner. The Consultant is not able to work with a Client who is angry, blaming, threatening and disrespectful.

* The Consultant puts his heart into his work and does his best to compassionately help the Client.

* The Consultant requires open and honest communication and always strives to give satisfying service.

* If the Client is dissatisfied with the Consultant's services and would like a monetary refund, the Consultant requires that the Client kindly notify the Consultant of this in a timely manner for a full and final release.

The Client agrees to:

* Make a full commitment to implement the healing and health-building guidelines detailed in *Self Healing Colitis & Crohn's* and those recommended by the Consultant, and to make this natural health approach his/her lifestyle with the goal of realizing a life of disease-free wellness.

* Study *Self Healing Colitis & Crohn's* on a daily basis until the information is fully understood and implemented on a daily routine basis.

* Set up the consultations, confirm each one and make the phone calls.

* Pay the Consultant for all of his questionnaire review and evaluation work, education and counseling work on the day of all rendered services.

* Work no more than four hours per day, only if necessary and physically possible and if the work is low-stress, and take a sabbatical with complete rest as soon as possible.

* Furnish copies of blood chemistry tests made within the last six months. If blood tests have not been conducted within the previous four weeks, have a new full panel of tests made, and submit a copy of the report to the Consultant.

* Keep a daily diary with diet, activity, health symptom and health condition details in e-mailable format, and provide updated diaries to the Consultant prior to consultations.

* Take full responsibility for his/her decisions and actions.

* Take full responsibility and the initiative for determining if he/she needs medical attention as the Consultant cannot make that determination since he is not a physician. The name(s) and phone number(s) of the Client's advising medical doctor(s) whom the Client will contact if medical attention is needed is/are as follows:

* Continue his/her health education during and after the healing phase. Additional recommended health education materials are available via the Consultant from his Living Nutrition's Health Mastery Catalog and from the Living Nutrition Online Bookstore at http://www.livingnutrition.com/bookstore. html.

Client: please sign your name indicating your understanding and agreement:

_____

Date _____

Please send a signed copy of this completed questionnaire to Dr. David Klein, Colitis & Crohn's Health Recovery Center, P.O. Box 256, Sebastopol, CA 95473 USA. Or fax it to (240) 414-5341. It is the client's responsibility to contact David Klein to set up consultations. Please phone (707) 829-0462 or (877) 740-6082 between 10:00 AM and 3:00 PM Pacific Standard Time, Monday through Thursday, or e-mail dave@colitis-crohns.com. I am looking forward to assisting you on your way to wellness!

C
HYGIENIC HEALTH CARE PROVIDERS

Center for Fruit Therapy
Lyudmila Emilova, M.D.
Varna, Bulgaria
www.emilova.org

Colitis and Crohn's Health Recovery Center
Dr. David Klein
Sebastopol, California
(877) 740-6082 or (707) 829-0462
www.colitis-crohns.com

Dr. Zarin Azar, Gastroenterologist
Los Angeles, California
(562) 402-2384

Fasting in Costa Rica With Dr. Douglas N. Graham
www.foodnsport.com
foodnsport@aol.com

TrueNorth Health Education Center
Dr. Allan Goldhamer
Santa Rosa, California
(707) 586-5555
www.healthpromoting.com

Vida Clara Fasting Retreat
Dr. Robert Sniadach
Belize
www.vidaclara.com

D
RECOMMENDED READING AND VIEWING

Some titles are available through the Living Nutrition Bookstore. Order online at www.livingnutrition.com/bookstore.html or call (707) 829-0462 or (877) 740-6082.

"Essential Natural Hygiene Course" and "Advanced Natural Hygiene Course." Sniadach, Dr. Robert W. Transformation Institute, School of Natural Hygiene. Baltimore, Maryland. 2006

"Fasting For Renewal." Shelton, Dr. Herbert M. American Natural Hygiene Society. Tampa, Florida. 1974

"Focusing." Gendlin, Ph.D., Eugene. Bantam Books. New York, New York. 1981

"Food Combining Made Easy." Shelton, Dr. Herbert M. Willow Publishing, Inc. San Antonio, Texas. 1997

"Fruit the Food and Medicine for Man." Krok, Morris. Essence of Health, Wandsbeck, South Africa. 1984

"Fruitarian Diet & Physical Rejuvenation." Abramowski, Dr. O. L. M. Living Nutrition Publications, Sebastopol, California. 2009.

"Grain Damage." Graham, Dr. Douglas N. The Cause of Health. Marathon, Florida. 1999

"High Energy Methods." Fry, T. C. Living Nutrition Publications, Sebastopol, California. 1997

"Living Nutrition and Vibrance Magazines." Living Nutrition Publications. Sebastopol, California

"Perfect Body." Roe Gallo, M. A., Roe Gallo Publishing. San Mateo, California. 2002

"Raw 'n Delish Vibrant Recipes." Living Nutrition Publications. Sebastopol, California. 2007

"Raw Vegetable Juices." Walker, D.Sci., N.W. The Berkeley Publishing Group. New York, New York. 1983

"Self Healing Power!" Fry, Dr. T. C., Shelton, Dr. Herbert, and Klein, David. Living Nutrition Publications. Sebastopol, California. 2002

"Superior Nutrition." Shelton, Dr. Herbert M. Willow Publishing, Inc. San Antonio, Texas. 1994

"The 80/10/10 Diet." Douglas N. Graham, D.C. FoodnSport Press. Key Largo, Florida. 2006

"The Art of Rejuvenation." Klein, Ph.D., David. Living Nutrition Publications. Sebastopol, California. 2007

"The China Study." Campbell, Ph.D., T. Colin and Campbell II, Thomas M. Ben Bella Books, Inc. Dallas, Texas. 2006

"The Diamond Approach." Davis, John. Shambhala Publications, Inc. Boston, Massachusetts. 1999

"The Essene Gospel of Peace." Szekely, Edmund Bordeaux. International Biogenic Society. Nelson, British Columbia, Canada. 1981

"The Fruits Of Healing—A Story About a Natural Healing of Ulcerative Colitis." Klein, David. Living Nutrition Publications. Sebastopol, California. 1999

"The High Energy Diet DVD." Graham, D.C., Douglas N. FoodNSport Press. Key Largo, Florida. 1990

"The New High Energy Diet Recipes." Graham, D.C., Douglas N. FoodNSport Press. Key Largo, Florida. 2007

"The Raw Food Pearamid and Food Combining Chart." Klein, David. Living Nutrition Publications. Sebastopol, California. 1997

"The Science and Fine Art of Food and Nutrition. The Hygienic System: Volume II." Shelton, Dr. Herbert M. American Natural Hygiene Society. Tampa, Florida. 1996

"The Science and Fine Art of Natural Hygiene. The Hygienic System, Volume I." Shelton, Dr. Herbert M. American Natural Hygiene Society. Tampa, Florida. 1996

"The Seven Spiritual Laws of Success." Chopra, M.D., Deepak. Amber-Allen Publishing. San Rafael, California. 1994

"The Undigestible Truth About Meat." Shaw, M.A., A.I.Y.S., Dr. Gina. GLS Publications. Clayhall, England. 2002

"The 80/10/10 Diet." Graham, Dr. Douglas N. FoodNSport Press. Key Largo, Florida. 2006

"Unlimited Power." Robbins, Anthony. Simon and Schuster. New York, New York. 1986

"Your Natural Diet: Alive Raw Foods." Fry, T. C. and Klein, David. Living Nutrition Publications. Sebastopol, California. 2002

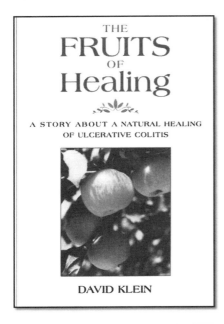

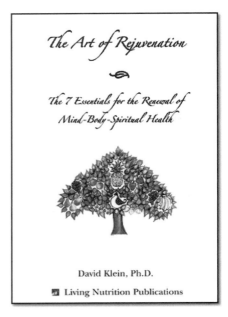

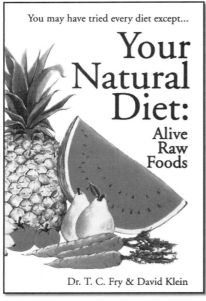

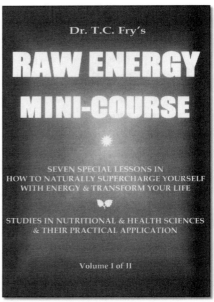

Order from Living Nutrition
Tel: (877) 740-6082
Online: www.livingnutrition.com

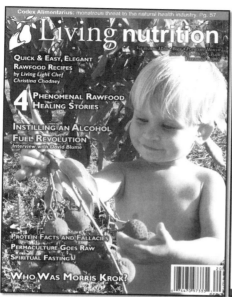

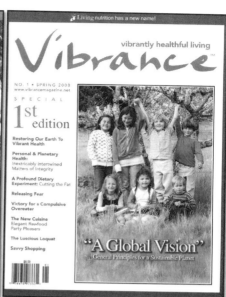

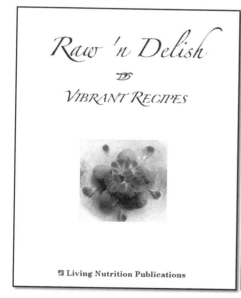

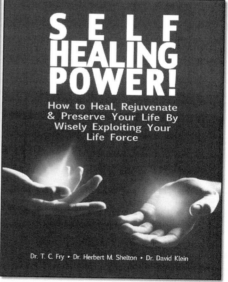

Order from Living Nutrition
Tel: (877) 740-6082
Online: www.livingnutrition.com

E
HEALTHFUL WEB SITES

Arnold's Way
www.arnoldsway.com

Breathing.com
www.breathing.com

Center for Fruit Therapy
www.emilova.org

Colitis & Crohn's Health Recovery Center
www.colitis-crohns.com

Diamond Logos Teachings
www.diamondlogos.com

DiscountJuicers.com
www.discountjuicers.com

Dr. Douglas N. Graham
www.foodnsport.com

Dr. Susan Smith Jones
www.susansmithjones.com

Fruitarian Worldwide Network
www.fruitnet.org

Health 101 Institute
www.health101.org

Living and Raw Food Community
www.living-foods.com

Living Nutrition and ***Vibrance Magazines,*** **Bookstore, Health Shop and Forum**
www.livingnutrition.com

OrganicAthlete
www.organicathlete.com

Raw 'n Delish Vibrant Recipes
www.rawndelish.us

Raw Passion
www.raw-passion.com

Ridhwan School—Diamond Approach Teachings
www.ridhwan.org

Self Healing Colitis & Crohn's
www.colitiscurebook.com

Self Healing Empowerment - Dr. David Klein's Home Page
www.selfhealingempowerment.com

Transformation Institute - School of Natural Hygiene
www.transformationinstitute.org

TrueNorth Health Education and Fasting Center
www.healthpromoting.com

University of Natural Health
www.unh-edu.org

UK Juicers
www.ukjuicers.com

Vegetarian USA
www.vegetarianusa.com

Vida Clara Fasting Retreat
www.vidaclara.com

F
REFERENCES

Baroody, N.D., D.C., Ph.D., Theodora A. "Alkalize or Die." Holographic Health Press. Waynesville, North Carolina. 1991

Balch, M.D., James F. and Balch, C.N.C., Phyllis A. "Prescription for Nutritional Healing." Avery Publishing Group. Garden City Park, New York. 1990

Bauman, M.Ed., Ph.D., Edward. "Nutrition and Your Health." Berkeley, California. 1984

California Avocado Commission. Irvine, California. www.avocado.org

Campbell, Ph.D., T. Colin and Campbell II, Thomas M. "The China Study." Ben Bella Books, Inc. Dallas, Texas. 2006

Cavaliere, Stephen and Post, Allison. "Unwinding the Belly." North Atlantic Books. Berkeley, California. 2003

Chopra, M.D., Deepak. "Ageless Body, Timeless Mind." Harmony Books. New York, New York. 1993

Clements, N.D., D.O., Harry. "Self-Treatment for Colitis." Thorsins Publishers. Wellingborough, England. 1978

Cousens, M.D., Gabriel. "Conscious Eating. Vision Books International. Mill Valley, California. 1992

Davis, John. "The Diamond Approach." Shambhala Publications, Inc. Boston, Massachusetts. 1999

Dong, A., Scott, S. C. "Serum Vitamin B_{12} and Blood Cell Values in Vegetarians." "The Annals of Nutrition and Metabolism vol. 26." University of Nutritional Sciences. University of Vienna. Vienna, Austria. 1982

Dorland, M.D., W. A. N. "Dorland's Illustrated Medical Dictionary 30th Edition." Elsevier-Health Sciences Division. Philadelphia, Pennsylvania. 2003

Doeser, Linda. "The Little Green Avocado Book." St. Martin's Press. New York, New York. 1981

Duke, J. "Handbook of Biologically Active Phytochemicals and Their Activities." CRC Press, Inc. Boca Raton, Florida. 1992

Ehret, Arnold. "Mucousless Diet Healing System." Ehret Literature Publishing Co. Dobbs Ferry, New York. 1983

Esser, Dr. William. "Dictionary of Natural Foods." Natural Hygiene Press. Bridgeport, Connecticut. 1972

Ford Heritage. "Composition and Facts About Foods." Health Research. Pomeroy, Washington. 1971

Fry, Marti. "Starches Are Second-rate Foods." "The Health Reporter, Volume 1, Report No. 3." Life Science Institute. Austin, Texas.

Fry, Dr. T. C. and Klein, David. "Your Natural Diet: Alive Raw Foods." Living Nutrition Publications. Sebastopol, California. 2004

Fry, T. C., Vetrano, Dr. Vivian V., et. al. "The Life Science Health System." Life Science Institute. Austin, Texas. 1986

Fullerton Arboretum. "California Rare Fruit Growers Inc. Fruit Facts, Volume One." California State University Fullerton. Fullerton, California. 1992

Goldstein, D.P.M., Jack. "Triumph Over Disease By Fasting." Arco Publishing Company. New York, New York. 1977

Graham, Dr. Douglas N. "Grain Damage." FoodnSport Press. Key Largo, Florida. 1998

Graham, Dr. Douglas N. "The 80-10-10 Diet." FoodnSport Press. Key Largo, Florida. 2006

Gray, Robert. "The Colon Health Handbook." Rockridge Publishing Co. Oakland, California. 1984

Great Smokies Diagnostic Laboratory. "Intestinal Permeability." Asheville, North Carolina. 1990 Guillory, M.D., Gerard. "IBS: A Doctor's Plan for Chronic Digestive Troubles." Hartley & Marks, Inc. Point Roberts, Washington. 1991

Guyton, M.D., Arthur C. "Anatomy and Physiology." Saunders College Publishing. New York, New York. 1985

Guyton and Hall, "Textbook of Medical Physiology, Eleventh Edition." Elsevier & Saunders. Philadelphia, Pennsylvania. 2005

Haas, M.D., Elson M. "Staying Healthy with Nutrition." Celestial Arts. Berkeley, California. 1992

Hartley-Hennessy, T. "Healing By Water or Drinking Sunlight and Oxygen." Essence of Health Publishing Co. Durban, South Africa. 1966

Hume, E. Douglas. "Béchamp or Pasteur?" Essence of Health Publishing Company. Westville, South Africa. 1976

Kime, Dr. Zane. "Sunlight." World Health Publications. Penryn, California. 1980

Klein, Ph.D., David. "Living Nutrition." Volumes 5, 13, 15. Living Nutrition Publications. Sebastopol, California. 1998, 2002, 2004

Klein, Ph.D., David. "Raw 'n Delish Vibrant Recipes." Living Nutrition Publications. Sebastopol, California. 2007

Klein, Ph.D., David. "The Art of Rejuvenation." Living Nutrition Publications. Sebastopol, California. 2007

Klein, David. "The Fruits of Healing, A Story About the Natural Healing of Ulcerative Colitis." Living Nutrition Publications. Sebastopol, California. 1999

Lay, N.D.,M.B.N.O.A., Joan. "Diets To Help Colitis." Thorsins Publishers. Wellingborough, England. 1980

Marieb, E., Hoehn, K. "Human Anatomy and Physiology." Pearson Education. Upper Saddle River, New Jersey. 2006

Mindell, Earl. "Vitamin Bible." Warner Books. New York, NY, 1981

Norman, Ph.D., Eric J. Norman Clinical Laboratory, Inc. Cincinnati, Ohio. Nov., 1999

Norris, J., R.D., "Vitamin B_{12}: Are You Getting It?" Vegan Outreach. Tuscon, Arizona. 2005

Peavy, W. and Peary, W. "Super Nutrition Gardening." Avery Publishing Group. New York, New York. 1993

Pratt, R., Johnson, E. "Journal of Pharmaceutical Sciences." Wiley-Liss, Inc. Hobpoken, New Jersey. 1968

Robbins, John. "The Diet Revolution." Conari Press. Berkeley, California. 2001

Shaw, Dr. Gina. M.A., A.I.Y.S. "The Undigestible Truth About Meat." GLS Publications. Clayhall, England. 2002

Shelton, Dr. Herbert M. "Food Combining Made Easy." Willow Publishing, Inc. San Antonio, Texas. 1997

Shelton, Dr. Herbert M. "Fasting Can Save Your Life." American Natural Hygiene Society. Tampa, Florida. 1999

Shelton, Dr. Herbert M. "Superior Nutrition." Willow Publishing, Inc. San Antonio, Texas. 1994

Shelton, N.D., D.C., Ph.D., Herbert M. "The Hygienic System. Vol. 1. Orthobionomics." Dr. Shelton's Health School. San Antonio, Texas. 1934

Shelton, Dr. Herbert M. "The Science and Fine Art of Food and Nutrition. The Hygienic System: Volume II." American Natural Hygiene Society. Tampa, Florida. 1996

Smith, C., Ph.D., Marks, A., M.D., Lieberman, M., Ph.D. "Marks' Basic Medical Biochemistry, Second Edition." Lippincott Williams & Wilkins. Hagerstown, Maryland. 2005

The Committee on Diet, Nutrition and Cancer. "Diet, Nutrition and Cancer." National Academy Press. Washington, D.C. 1982

USDA. "USDA Nutrient Database for Standard Reference, Release 13, November, 1999." www.nal.usda.gov.

Van den Berg, H., Dagnelie, P.C., van Staveren, W.A. "Vitamin B_{12} and Seaweed." "The Lancet." London, England. Jan. 30, 1988

Vander, Sherman, Lucino. "Human Physiology." McGraw-Hill, New York, New York. 1994

Walker, D.Sci., N.W. "Raw Vegetable Juices." The Berkeley Publishing Group. New York, New York, 1983

Walsh, S., Ph.D. "What Every Vegan Should Know About Vitamin B_{12}." www.beyondveg.com/walsh-s/vitamin-b12/vegans-1.shtml. 2001

Watanabe, F., Katsura, H., Takenaka, S., Fujita, T., Abe, K., Tamura, Y., Nakatsuka, T., Nakano, Y. "Pseudovitamin B_{12} is the predominant cobamide of an algal health food, spirulina tablets." Journal of Agricultural and Food Chemistry. Davis, California. Nov., 1999

Weinberger, C.M.T., Stanley, "Healing Within." Published by Beth Kuper. Mill Valley, California. 1993

Lashner, L.A., et al. "Passive Smoking is Associated With an Increased Risk of Developing Inflammatory Bowel Disease in Children." "Gastroenterology." Elsevier, Inc. New York, New York. April, 1992

Williams, Sue Rodwell. "Essentials of Nutrition and Diet Therapy." Times Mirror/Mosby College Publishing. St. Louis, Missouri. 1990

G

ABOUT THE AUTHOR

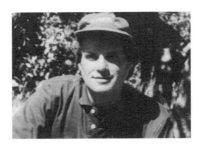

Dr. David Klein has been Director of the Colitis & Crohn's Health Recovery Center, currently located in Sebastopol in northern California, since 1993.

Dr. Klein is a Hygienic Doctor with a Ph.D. in Natural Health and Healing and a certified Nutrition Educator. Dr. Klein's approach is wholistic and is based upon Natural Hygiene, the world's most successful health science program over the last 200 years. Since 1992, Dr. Klein has counseled over 2,000 clients back to health via the principles of Natural Hygiene and he has taught nutrition classes and given health and nutrition lectures. Dr. Klein's own unique healing journey, his studies of many disciplines of health science, and his extensive professional experience have given him uncommon insight into the requisites of healing and health by which he is able to consistently guide people from disease to rejuvenation.

Dr. Klein is also Editor of *Living Nutrition* and *Vibrance Magazines,* the world's most-read raw food lifestyle magazines. Dr. Klein is also a Professor with the new University of Natural Health (see www.livingnutrition.com/university. html). Dr. Klein's book *Your Natural Diet: Alive Raw Foods* is the text for the course "Humans' Natural Biological Diet."

Dr. Klein is on the Board of Directors as a nutritional and healing advisor for St. John's Colonic Center in Bowie, Maryland (colonics are not recommended for inflammatory bowel disease). His book *Self Healing Colitis & Crohn's* is used as the teaching model for a course taught at the Canadian School of Natural Nutrition. He has led Raw Passion seminars over the last 10 years and co-produced Rawstock health festivals in northern California.

Dr. Klein has thrived on a 100% vegan diet of mostly raw foods since 1984. Originally from New Jersey, he also holds a B.S. in civil engineering and worked 10 years in the field of environmental engineering before starting his health education businesses and practice. Leading people to health independence is Dr. Klein's passion.

Dr. David Klein's Web Sites

- www.colitis-crohns.com
- www.colitiscurebook.com
- www.selfhealingempowerment.com
- www.livingnutrition.com
- www.rawndelish.us
- www.raw-passion.com
- www.rawstock.us
- www.fruitnet.org

Self-published Works By Dr. David Klein

- *Living Nutrition* and *Vibrance Magazines*
- *Raw 'n Delish Vibrant Recipes*
- *Self Healing Colitis & Crohn's*
- *Self Healing Power!* by Dr. T. C. Fry, Dr. Herbert Shelton and David Klein
- *The Art of Rejuvenation*
- *The Fruits Of Healing - A Story About a Natural Healing of Ulcerative Colitis*
- *Your Natural Diet: Alive Raw Foods* by Dr. T. C. Fry & David Klein

Dr. David Klein's Abbreviated Healing Story

My journey into the health education field began in 1975, when at age 17 my robust health began to gradually decline. A heavy eater of meat and junk food, my physical and mental energies deteriorated over a period of six months, then I experienced incessant diarrhea. After a few weeks of medical treatment, I showed little improvement, so a colon examination was done. The diagnosis was ulcerative colitis, and I spent my 18th birthday in a hospital, taking prednisone and azulfadine drug treatments. The symptoms subsided, temporarily, but the drugs further ruined my health and had a devastating effect on my mental abilities.

Within a few months, feeling sickly and very weak, I experienced a recurrence of the diarrhea and additional symptoms, including cramping and bleeding, and this led to further physical deterioration. What ensued were eight tortuous years of colitis flare-ups and off-and-on drug therapy. At age 26, after eight years of ulcerative colitis while attending engineering school followed by working in the environmental engineering field, I was reduced to a weak, sickly shadow of my former self. I was having gastric eruptions every time I ate and up to 10 painful bowel movements a day with mucous and blood. My gut always hurt, my nervous system became shattered and I experienced hellish nightmares as I was toxic, debilitated by the medicines, severely demineralized and over-stressed by my diet and medicines. I was no longer able to work or leave my house.

Although my life had become a dying hell, I never gave in to the medical doctors' advice to accept my illness and just be patient until their impossible "miracle drug cure" came along; I desperately wanted my health back and doubted that the doctors knew what they were doing.

In 1984, I had the great fortune to find a nutritionist and Doctor of Natural Hygiene, Dr. Laurence Galant in Staten Island. He introduced me to the concepts of self-healing and eating a fruit-based diet and he gave me Natural Hygiene literature to study. At first I thought the idea of eating mostly fruit while having nonstop diarrhea was crazy. Yet, I studied Natural Hygiene literature and slowly cleaned up my diet. I was attached to eating chicken and other favorite cooked foods, however, and was still having colitis flare-ups and relying on medicines.

In the fall of 1984 I had a colonoscopy exam which confirmed that I had advanced ulcerations throughout my sick colon. Surmising that I had been chronically sick and was not getting better and would eventually face cancer, the gastroenterologist recommended that I either try his experimental drug, which knocks out the immune system, or have my colon surgically removed. Upon hearing this, a heavy decisive thought entered my mind: "I have had it with this medical madness—I'll be dead soon if I don't find the answer myself!" I recognized that my life was a gradual descent into hell and I had to climb out now because it was almost too late.

Over the next few days I started thinking like never before about how to overcome my illness. I realized that I had to figure out what the MD's could not, and my thinking led me to consider more closely the information on self-healing and switching to a vegan diet. The information seemed so incredible, but I saw that it was really working for Dr. Galant, and I had read many amazing healing testimonials.

Then one amazing night while studying Dr. T. C. Fry's Life Science/Natural Hygiene course, I beheld a healing vision and it all made sense; the picture of my new health was revealed via the Natural Hygiene healthful living system. I understood that humans are biologically fruit eaters and that fruit was the best food for my sick colon and entire body. I was ecstatic knowing I had solved the diet mystery, conquered the myths about humans' natural diet and the care of disease and set myself free!

The next day I threw away the medicines, divorced myself from all medical intervention for good, gave up all meat and dairy forever and started a three-day fresh-made juice diet. By the second day I was coming back to life. On the third day I was feeling better and better and my enthusiasm and joy drove my family crazy! My gut was feeling soothed, I was rejuvenating and the nightmarish illness was over. On the fourth day, upon adding solid fruits including bananas to my diet, I had solid stools and greatly diminished symptoms. I had set myself free of illness, doctors and medicines for good, and my bowels were working better and better with no signs of toxicity!

I adopted a fruit-based, vegan diet—that harmonized best with my mind/body/spirit. And with that my energies continuously increased as I detoxified and began rebuilding. Within about four to six weeks I felt that my colon was completely healed. I was able to enjoy eating and living again. With my bowels functioning better than ever, I began a new active healthful lifestyle.

Over the next few years I diligently worked at rebuilding my depleted body, incorporating daily running and yoga, all the while studying the life sciences and all of the physical, mental, emotional and spiritual factors which determine our health. It took several years of total dedication to build robust health. In 1993, after a year of study and training at the Institute for Educational Therapy in Cotati, California (now known as Bauman College in Penngrove, California), I became certified as a Nutrition Educator and began providing nutrition and healing consultations. In 2006 I received a Ph.D./Hygienic Doctor degree in Natural Health and Healing from the University of Natural Health. *Self Healing Colitis and Crohn's* served as my thesis. Today, at age 51, I enjoy excellent dynamic health and vitality.

Healing is easy if we understand and apply the principle that it is the body that does the healing. When we remove the unhealthful aspects of our diet and lifestyle and step out of the way, the body will do the healing work automatically and naturally.

Living healthfully is the easiest and most joyful way to be, and I am glad to help health seekers get there and feel that for themselves. Each of us deserves glorious health!